GIVE BIRTH
WITHOUT FEAR

SUSANNA HELI

GIVE BIRTH WITHOUT FEAR

PRACTICAL TOOLS FOR A CONFIDENT BIRTH

ISBN: 978-91-987910-0-6
Also available as an ebook, ISBN 978-91-987910-1-3

Contents

Introduction

THOUGHT I KNEW MY BODY and that I was well-prepared to give birth. I could not have been more wrong! I could never have imagined what giving birth was going to be like, the unforeseeable force that rushed through my body, and how much it frightened me. The pain was not at all what I had imagined it was going to be like, and I was shocked by its enormous power. Suddenly, I did not want to give birth at all! I started to fight my own body. I tried to talk to it, begging it to stop. I just wanted to get away, to escape, to disappear. Without me realising it, the fear took over completely.

I was terrified of everything; I was terrified when a contraction started and also when it ended, since that meant a new one was on its way! I dreaded the pain and felt that I would not have the stamina to see this process through. Mostly, I was fearing for my life, without really knowing why. Fear had taken over my whole being and was blocking everything else out.

In the midst of all this struggle, my partner tells me my midwife, Cayenne Ekjordh, wants to talk to me over the phone. I yell at him, tell him I do not want to talk to anyone. Despite this, he puts the receiver to my ear. Her words flow out of the speaker, telling me I am only making it worse by hyperventilating and tensing my body – which I was not even aware that I was doing. She tells me I have two choices; I can keep on doing what I am doing and have a very difficult birth, or I can choose to listen to her. This was not a difficult choice to make; I start listening.

She helps me to breathe in a new way, softly and quietly, and tells me to let my body become *heavy* during the contractions and to simply let the birth happen. She says that I need to relax and follow my body, instead of tensing up and resisting its lead. Slowly, I start to listen to her, and I stop fighting. Despite the fear, I let my body become heavy and my breath soften when each contraction begins. The contrast is so amazing that I decide, in that moment, to start trusting my body, that it knows what it is doing and that I have everything it takes to give birth to my baby.

This new attitude towards my own body turned out to make all the difference, and it opened up a new world for me. I realised that by letting go of fear, I could suddenly tune in to my body and help it to give birth. It did not, in any way, make the process easy and it did not take away the pain. It did, however, help me find my way back to my body, which, in turn, knew how to give birth. I was able to use various movements, breathing, relaxation, sound and the power of the mind in the form of positive images and words. These simple tools gave me the strength to face the pain and fear, and I gave birth to my son a few hours later.

After birthing him, I realised I would probably have continued to hyperventilate and tense my whole body had I not been helped to find the way back to breathing silently and relaxing down in the contractions. I would never have known the difference that this could make, and I would have assumed that the panic I felt was part of the birth process. This insight was so profound that it made me want to help others find this inner power.

I started working as an assistant nurse on a labour ward. I soon noticed a lot of women experiencing the same fear I had felt during labour. *Again and again*, I saw women showing signs of extreme physical distress caused by fear when facing pain. Pain led to fear,

fear led to stress, and stress led to negative physical reactions, blocking the body by activating the fight-or-flight response and the stress system. The women were extremely tense, they hyperventilated and could focus only on the pain. Their shoulders were up high, their jaws were clenched, their voices sounded panicked, and they could neither rest nor sleep. As for me the fear blocked them completely, draining their focus and strength.

I started to use the simple tools I had used with my son in order to break or shift the negative pattern the women were trapped in. Time and time again, I witnessed how women, with the help of these simple tools, were able to change the fight-or-flight response and give birth without fear. I understood then that it was not the *pain* itself, it was actually *fear* that was the cause of the stress reactions blocking the body. Suddenly, with the help of the tools, the women could handle the fear and cope with the birthing process in a different way. The contractions were no less challenging, but the pain became less frightening, and the women were able to find something within themselves – an inner power helping them to give birth.

The modern health care system seemed to have forgotten the key foundation of how to help women handle the contractions with the help of breathing, relaxation, the voice and the power of the mind, and I was amazed to discover their remarkable effects. These simple tools were an important missing piece of the puzzle, enabling women to get in touch with their inner ability to give birth. I realised that I wanted to work with the *emotional aspects* of childbirth, rather than the medical part. I wanted to make sure women did not just have a medically safe birth, but equally an emotionally safe birth.

Along with working as an assisting nurse, I started working as a doula – a support person for women in childbirth. In order to get a deeper understanding of how the emotions impact the body and the physiology of birth, I chose to go to university to become a psychosomatic physiotherapist – a physiotherapist working with the mind–body connection. Many years and hundreds of births later, I have written the book *Give Birth Without Fear* and created the Birth Without Fear method.

The book was first published in Sweden 2009 and has since then helped thousands of women and their partners and support persons to have an emotionally safe birth. The method is used by the healthcare system to lessen stress and fear before and during childbirth to prevent traumas and negative birth experiences. Today the home of the book and method in different languages is our global mother organisation 'Birth By Heart' (www. birthbyheart.com).

The book consists of *three* parts. The first section gives you necessary knowledge about, and a deeper understanding of, how we *react* to fear and stress, and what is important in order to deal with these feelings. To be able to work against fear, it is necessary to understand the opposite feelings of trust and confidence, but also the purpose of pain in the normal birth process.

The second part of the book is the concrete and *practical* part. Here, I introduce the four tools of the 'Birth Without Fear method': breathing, relaxation, the voice and the power of the mind and how you can use them in the contractions. I then explain how you can use the tools during the different phases of childbirth, with or without pain relief, as well as the importance of both resting and being active.

To prevent fear, and to use the tools, you also need *support* during childbirth. Therefore, the third part of the book deals with the importance of support. Receiving support during childbirth is important, whether you are in a relationship or not. You can get this support from a partner, a friend, a doula or a family member. This is why I have chosen to call the person who adopts this role the 'support person'. This part of the book is aimed both at you and your support person, and includes information, advice and instructions about what is important when supporting a woman during labour. This section also looks at the power of touch and massage.

The book ends with a short *summary* of all the techniques and instructions; it can be used as a quick reference guide for you and your support person.

You can use 'The Birth Without Fear method' and the tools in this book whether you give birth vaginally, by assisted birth or by caesarean section; no matter whether you choose to have some form of pain relief or not; whether everything is straightforward or there are complications. They work at home, in the hospital or in a midwifery led unit. This is because regardless of where or how you give birth, it is your birth and you still need support and the ability to handle what may unfold. By using the tools in this book, you can assist your body and experience an inner strength and a positive childbirth, no matter what the external circumstances may be.

I wrote this book to help you handle the fear that can surface during childbirth, so that it does not block your ability to give birth. I use the word 'fear' to encapsulate negative emotions, such as doubt, meaninglessness, dejection, feelings of anxiety and aggression. These emotions can hinder the body from accessing its inner ability by triggering negative chain reactions, such as the fight-or-flight response.

I do not think it is possible to always give birth entirely without fear. However, by using the tools in this book you will be able to minimise the fear and take control of it. When fear no longer seizes all your focus and energy, you will be able to feel more secure, more involved in the process, and less scared. When the body *ceases* to perceive a *threat*, the pain will ease and become less destructive. When fear is no longer blocking the body, the uterus can do its work and the birth process can advance and you will be able to access the amazing inherited ability to give birth you already have inside.

My wish is that this book will help you feel more present, participatory and strong during your labour, and that it gives you the confidence to give birth. Remember that all women are unique and all birth experiences different. There is no right or wrong way to give birth. Discover what may work the best for you and use the book to inspire you to trust and listen to your body. Let go of all your preconceptions about giving birth. Be open minded. Be brave and respect yourself. Seek the wisdom your body already possesses. This inner voice only wants one thing – to help you give birth to your baby.

Good luck!
With love! Susanna Heli

1

Confident birth

The human body is an amazing instrument and you already have all the knowledge you need to give birth to your baby. Fear, however, can get in the way of the body accessing this knowledge. This is because fear activates stress reactions, which are essentially designed to keep you out of harm's way. This is an ancient mechanism which has been crucial for the survival of our species. However, since we no longer encounter the same threatening situations as we used to, this mechanism can get in the way of the birthing process.

Most of this manifestation takes place without you being aware of it, which makes it more challenging to do something about. It is possible though to interrupt, divert and prevent this negative spiral. In this section, you will learn to understand fear, where it comes from, how it affects you, and how to break its cycle. When fear no longer swallows up all your focus and energy, you will be free to access the power within you – the power that will help you to give birth.

Understanding fear

During labour, you and your body connect in a special way. You face your most basic instincts, which you might never have encountered before, or at least not very often in your life so far. You leave behind the day-to-day world you know and enter into a new dimension which may be unfamiliar, but where your body knows exactly what to do. This is natural and part of the physiological heritage your body carries within; you are made to do this. However, this does not automatically make childbirth easy. The enormous physical work that is unfolding inside you is unlike anything you have ever previously faced, and therefore it can feel unnatural compared to what you experience in your everyday life.

To be able to overcome fear, it is important to comprehend and understand the purpose of pain in the natural and healthy birth progresses, and what takes place in your body during the various stages of this normal process. Therefore, this part will teach you more about how the body is built. However, in order to differentiate between reactions caused by the natural process of birthing, as opposed to reactions caused by fear, you will need to know how the body reacts to fear. Sometimes, you do not understand what reaction leads to another, which can create even more fear. You might think the physical chaos you are experiencing is synonymous with labour, when in fact it is actually a response to fear. Understanding these feelings and learning how to influence the stress cycle will help you to avoid this pitfall. This is why we now together are going to explore what fear is, why it has such power over us today, and why it can cause problems during childbirth.

Childbirth – a journey within

Fear is a natural and fundamental feeling, which helps us to survive. However, there is a big difference between the fear women experience today and the fear women have experienced throughout history. Since modern, Western maternity care is one of the medically safest in the world, we worry less about illnesses, complications or death during childbirth. Nevertheless, many people working within maternity care today agree that for many women the fear of childbirth is rising, and that this fear can influence the birthing process in a negative way. This increase in fear has led to more and more women requesting planned caesarean sections, and there are more women who experience posttraumatic stress disorder (PTSD) and who need birth trauma counselling after labour and the birth of their baby.

Despite the high level and standard of medical care women receive today – alongside the fact that women today are more prepared than ever before, many reading widely about giving birth – they are more afraid than ever. Somewhere in the mix of new technology and promises of a pain-free existence, we have lost something fundamental. Despite the safe medical care, all the technological advances and information available, many women feel that something is missing – another kind of knowledge, a knowledge that will help them trust in their own body's ability and prepare for childbirth.

You may be thinking that you do not feel scared of giving birth, and that this does not apply to you. Fear can have a strong presence during pregnancy, but it can also spring up unexpectedly during childbirth. Of course, it is possible that you will not be scared either before, during, or after childbirth. However, I believe most women do experience fear at some point during birth, and that this is normal. The birthing process is both an extreme and intense experience, and it is therefore not surprising that different emotions come and go. Fear is just one of these emotions. However, if you do not understand what you are feeling, fear can escalate uncontrollably and block your body's ability to give birth. Therefore, it is very important to understand how fear might affect you, both physically and emotionally. If you really understand how your body reacts to fear, you will be able to apply the four tools presented in the next section, which will swiftly break or lessen the feeling of fear.

Labour and birth can be compared to preparing for a hike up a mountain; you assume you will enjoy the walk, that you will be able to complete the journey, that it will give you pleasure and you look forward to the feeling you will get after the completed challenge. Before setting off you will have prepared yourself for what to do on the journey and also considered what equipment you will need in the event of any unexpected situations arising.

You can apply the exact same mindset to giving birth. The birth is your hike into your inner landscape, and this book is your map. You assume that this journey is going to both challenge and strengthen you, that you have the ability to give birth, and that there will be a lot of joy at the end of the journey. However, you have also prepared for the unexpected 'storms' that might arise. You know that a 'storm' can be a huge challenge, but also that storms come and go – you just need to know how to weather them. If you get lost, you will, with the right tools and inner preparation, easily be able to re-track your way back to experience the joy of childbirth.

Ancient survival mechanism

In order to answer the question *why* fear can become a problem during childbirth, we need to look far back in history. Humankind has gone through enormous changes within a very short time. Today, many of the threatening situations our ancestors might have encountered are gone. Mentally, we have mostly learned to adapt to these changes, but our bodies still carry the automatic reaction patterns. Our emotions play an important part as messengers, which in turn trigger chain reactions. Every emotion has its own unique, bodily expression, and its own unique function.

Fear is an alarm signal preparing the body to react when facing potential threats – this is the fight-or-flight response. The emotion acts as a red alert mechanism, mobilising the body to meet the challenges or threatening situations ahead. The body prioritises the fear impulse over the ongoing birth, since survival is always of most importance. Stress hormones rush through our bloodstream to give us a boost of energy and sharpen our focus. Our attention increases, our vigilance sharpens, our pupils widen, the reproductive system slows down, our muscles get a rush of extra blood and the respiratory system speeds up to maximise the flow of oxygen. Stress reactions caused by fear can be simplified as a physiological 'No!' to birth. The body receives information about a potential threat and blocks itself in order to slow down the birthing process.

It all makes perfect sense if you look at this response from an evolutionary perspective. If our ancient ancestors found themselves in a situation where they were being chased by a bear or other wild animal, or they were in the midst of a war or battle, it was important for them to be able to flee during labour, without giving birth to the baby whilst on the run.

Problems arise when the threat you are facing comes from *within your own body*, like if you get scared of the pain or the physical work the body has to go through in order to birth the baby. In this case, the cause of the stress reaction does not go away, since its origin is internal, compared to when the threat originates from exterior circumstances. The body's response is to block labour, but fear no longer has a valid purpose. The body does not understand that there is no outer threat. It only responds to the *sensation* and *emotion* of fear, which is primarily designed as a warning and alarm system.

Fear not only has an effect on your *body*, but also on your *emotions* and your *mind*. In order to help you locate the threat, tunnel vision sets in, which helps you focus on the danger you are facing. This means that pain gets all the attention. Everything else ceases to exist, except for the sensation of pain, as it dominates over all other emotions and feelings. If this stress reaction is prolonged, with no time for recovery, it will eventually trigger feelings of hopelessness and negative emotions will be given free rein.

I have seen many labouring women enter negative stress patterns. When I help them to break free from these stress patterns, the experience of childbirth suddenly shifts and they can experience a much wider range of feelings and sensations. They can laugh, sleep, listen to their bodies, cuddle with their partner and many other things. Labour changes from a stressful, negative event, into a challenge that they can handle.

The body as messenger

Why is it that we are afraid of something that is so fundamental, and which is safer now than ever before? Today we generally see labour as a medical matter, rather than as an important life event that allows us to develop emotionally. Our lives revolve more and more around our external surroundings, as opposed to what is happening inside us. Work, careers and our impossibly complicated lives steal more and more of our attention. The body and its functions have time and time again been reduced to something irritating and troublesome. We no longer see them as having any meaning, or as something important. Today, for example, we regard pain as negative, and we believe a life without it is a human right. We do not stop to listen and learn when we feel pain. Often, we see pain as something that gets in our way; it hinders and bothers us in our effort to live our lives the way we want to. We no longer ask *why* we get stomach pain, headaches or muscular pain, or even why our whole body is full of pain; instead, we simply take a pill, or go and see the doctor. Neither have we learned that we are capable of handling pain and challenges in life, that they pass and that we actually can grow from them.

This attitude can be problematic during labour. Suddenly, you cannot simply *erase* the bodily signals or the pain. They demand your attention. You are thrown into an extreme, physical experience and you are expected to know how to deal with it, and how to act. All this is expected of you, without you having learned to trust the fact that pain has an important function and that your body has the *capacity* to handle it.

Your body knows how to give birth, however, if we do not view the body and its functions and signals as meaningful, it becomes something alien and dangerous, which in turn creates a separation between us and our own body. The pain of labour might then be experienced as an external force that takes over the body, leaving you more or less helpless. You are reacting to what happens inside you as if it were an external threat, in turn making you feel scared and triggering the fight-or-flight response. The fear tells your body, 'You are not allowed to go into labour now, there is a potential threat!' At this point, the body puts the 'brakes' on the whole birthing process, potentially causing it to become more drawn out and more painful.

It is therefore necessary to actively build confidence in the body's ability, and to collect all the knowledge needed about how to facilitate the birthing process. Regardless if you use pain relief or not. By understanding what is happening and the meaning of your body's signals and the pain, you will start to feel that your body is no longer something alien, but that you understand and work together with your own body. Your body and your mind can become one entity, working towards a common goal – giving birth to your baby!

Exercise

Listen to Your Body

You will never be able to predict exactly what is going to happen during labour. Instead, it is important to accept everything that occurs, by getting to know your thoughts and feelings. Practice listening to what your body is telling you. Notice the changes, such as a growing belly, the baby moving around, the pelvis aching, or some other sensation you might experience. The signals might not be that easy to distinguish at first and might be hard to define, but with practice it will get easier and easier to put what you are experiencing into words.

1. Position yourself comfortably. Turn off all sounds and lights. Make sure you are wearing something comfortable. Close your eyes.
2. Focus on your thoughts. Direct your attention towards what is happening inside of you right now. What thoughts and emotions emerge? Notice them for a while. Observe both negative and positive thoughts without judgement. Observe simply 'Here comes a thought or a feeling...'
3. Notice your feelings. What emotions are you filled with right now? Accept all your feelings, even the ones you do not wish to currently feel, such as difficult or unpleasant ones. Also welcome the ones that are pleasant, positive, lovely and exciting. Let feelings come and go without dwelling on them. Do not look for reasons as to how or why they are there. Your feelings are not who you are; simply let them be.

4. Welcome your body's signals. Then, do the same with your body's sensations. How does your body feel? Tense? Does it hurt? Is it itchy? Relaxed? Do not judge or evaluate, but simply notice what you are experiencing.

5. Now that you are more or less in the present moment, you should focus all your attention on one single sensation: *your breath*. Pay attention to what your inhalations and exhalations feel like through your body. Focus on one thing at a time, for example, how your stomach moves.

6. Then, let your thoughts expand; whilst staying aware of your breath, pay attention to your whole body, from your feet, up to your head. At the same time as you are aware of your breath and your body, become aware of your thoughts and feelings. You are one with your breath, your body, your feelings and your thoughts. Your breath has become something more; you now breathe with your entire body and your senses. They are all part of one whole.

Your experience is as important as medical safety

Contrary to popular belief, a positive or a negative birth experience is not determined by the kind of pain relief used, where the birth takes place, or any complications or external circumstances that might arise. Instead, it is the ability to handle any emotions and fears that might arise during labour, that plays a vital part of your experience.

When I first started working as a doula, I thought my job was to help women have the 'perfect birth'. If complications arose during birth, I felt like a failure and I thought the women would be dissatisfied. Instead, they were very pleased and felt empowered after giving birth and saw the experience, on the whole, as a positive one. During their entire labour they had felt acknowledged and that their feelings had been taken seriously. They had felt they could handle the fear. Importantly, this is what had given them the positive experience.

This also explains why some women who seemingly experience a very smooth and uncomplicated birthing process, still reflect on it as an extremely negative event. It is often the *feelings* of *fear* and *anxiety*, alongside the inability to deal with these feelings, that creates this negative experience. The Birth Without Fear method's purpose and task is therefore to *protect the labour experience*, rather than to try to facilitate the 'perfect birth'.

The inability to handle feelings of fear and anxiety during labour can not only activate stress reactions and block the body's abilities to birth, it can also impact life beyond birth in different ways. It can lead to depression, fear of future pregnancies, low self-confidence, a distrust in the workings of your body, nightmares, PTSD and difficulties bonding with your baby. With these consequences in mind, feelings of panic and extreme fear should be seen as a severe complication during labour, and everything possible should be done to try to avoid or minimise these feelings.

Many women feel they lack the inner strategies and tools needed to meet the challenges and feelings they might encounter during labour. Women are also often shocked to discover there is little or no help available to deal with these issues on maternity wards. However, maybe it is not the responsibility of the maternity wards to provide this type of care. It may be that we have come to a point where we need to look within ourselves in order to discover what we are missing. What if the solution is not out there, but is instead inside of you? What if you – *if you only knew how* – could realise that you have all the power and trust you need already within you? Your body is designed to give birth and will show you the way, if you only find the way to listen to it.

Pain relief or no pain relief?

Many people wonder if pain medication is enough when dealing with pain and fear. I am often asked if I am for or against drugs during labour; do I think it is good or bad to use them, is it natural or unnatural? I have been present at births taking place both at hospitals and within people's homes. I have been present at births where women have had pain relief and those without, as well as being present at caesarean births. Some births have had a lot of complications, whilst many have had no complications at all. What I have learned after all these years is what I mentioned above, that it is the *inner*, rather than the *outer* circumstances, that determine if a birth ends up being a positive or a negative experience.

Questions about pros and cons when it comes to pain relief are too complex and nuanced to cover in this book, and there are no straightforward answers. Medical interventions should not be seen as an easy way out; all of them can have side effects and it is important to know about them. One woman I assisted as a doula described the decision as to whether or not to take pain relief as swapping one bad thing for another. There are times when the advantages do outweigh the disadvantages when it comes to using pain relief during labour, since not all natural births are without complications.

What is important when making the decision is that you do not decide to use drugs *because of your fear*, or because you think that they will eliminate all pain. Scientific research points out that the reason many women are using pain relief is because they are afraid. The same research also shows that many of these women still find labour to be a negative, painful and frightening experience. From this, we can conclude that pain relief does not necessarily take away feelings of anxiety and fear. Medications will help take the edge off the pain if it becomes too overwhelming, and it can serve as a necessary complement to make the birthing process a bit easier.

However, in order to handle your feelings during labour, you also need something else; you need to learn *how* to manage them, and you need *tools* and *support*. The strategies within this book will help you through the birthing process and give you the ability to experience your own unique birth as a positive journey. It is importantly *how you experience the birth*, rather than how the birth went, that will impact your confidence, as well as influence whether or not you will want to give birth again. Therefore, managing your feelings is more important for your experience of giving birth than any type of pain medication.

Anita's Birth Story

I was searching for knowledge, a method and strength. Memories of my first son's birth brought feelings of fear, anxiety, pain and humiliation. With a few months to go until my next birth, I realised I did not want to go through the same hellish experience again, ever. I was convinced there had to be another way, with more support and better help to be able to understand how to let go during birth. I got in touch with a midwife, but our conversations did not give me the guidance I needed. Eventually, I got them from the four tools described in this book. They led to the birth of my second son being a fantastic experience.

I started to feel the early contractions in the evening, but I went to bed with a calm and easy mind. I felt ready. During the night I was woken up by the first contractions, and I managed to rely on the relaxation techniques I had been practicing for several months. I had forgotten the paralysing pain experienced in my previous birth; instead, by focusing on breathing softly and quietly, I was able to sleep in between contractions. I got up around 5 am and felt that I was more able to handle the contractions. The relaxation and breathing exercises (the soft, wonderful breathing) helped me focus and follow my body's lead. I remembered not to fight the contractions, nor to stiffen up in fear of the next one.

I kept busy by baking, and I met each irregular contraction by closing my eyes and standing upright, with my knees slightly bent and my arms hanging loose. I repeated a mantra to myself to make me focus my energy down towards the floor and make me feel heavy. When my eyebrows started to pull up and tense, my partner firmly and slowly stroked downwards on my arms and back.

We had breakfast and the force of my contractions intensified. It felt liberating to end the contraction with a great, big sigh to welcome the break. I had to stand up when I received the contractions now, but I could handle them without fear or panic. My partner had to remind me to breathe, as the sweat started flowing and we both felt it was time to leave.

We got to the delivery room and my partner was my primary focus. I kept close to him, as he talked me through the contractions, which were now coming more and more frequently. He encouraged me to relax my brow, my shoulders to sink, and he reminded me to breathe quietly. I became aware of how I could work WITH my body, and I was actually not scared of the pain.

The waters broke with a splash, and the force of the bearing-down contractions made me lose control. The mantra was gone. The mindfulness of what I was doing was also gone. The only things that felt real were my partner's touch and voice. I had somehow managed to undress, and after some more contractions, the baby came. With him came the release, the happiness, the joy, and the rush of knowing that this time, I was able to access my inner power and my body in an unbelievably radical way.

Handling the fear

Your body already knows how to give birth. Many generations before you have given birth, and that wisdom is partly programmed inside of you. The birthing process is a result of thousands of years of evolution, where Mother Nature, through her fantastic ability to create the optimal circumstances, has found this way for us to give birth. Everything is thoroughly thought out, down to the very smallest of details.

Specific physiological changes need to take place for a baby to be born. The cervix (the neck of the womb) needs to open, and the muscles of the uterus (the womb) need to contract and relax rhythmically for the baby to be able to pass down through the pelvis. These transitions require effort, and women experience them with varying degrees of pain. However, you are fully equipped to handle these changes as long as you allow them to happen. Therefore, try your very best to trust your body, with or without pain medication.

While childbirth is a completely natural, bodily process, it is also one of the greatest emotional and physical challenges a woman can go through. Your ability to handle emotions and obstacles will be put to the test. During labour, order will mix with chaos, and joy will meet pain. You might experience childbirth as something positive, exciting and challenging, or as something terrifying, chaotic and threatening. All of these emotions can be present during the same birth, and many women are not quite prepared for this emotional paradox. To prepare for this experience you will need to find an inner strength to handle positive as well as negative emotions during labour.

Coping

According to Aaron Antonovsky – a professor of medical sociology who has done a lot of research on stress – it is the feeling of *comprehensibility, manageability* and *meaningfulness* that makes it easier for us to handle life's challenges. These three components sum up the inner capability to see life as it is, and they are crucial when determining how you handle successes, as well as setbacks. Childbirth is one of those challenges in life where your general attitude and your life experiences will play an important part.

Fear and stress arise when you feel that your ability to handle what is in front of you does not meet the perceived expectations of what you should be able to handle. In as early as the 1960s, Richard Lazarus – an American researcher on stress – showed that it is the individual's *interpretation* of a given situation that determines the stress reaction, and not the situation itself. This is called *coping*. Coping is about the inner (thoughts and emotions) and outer (tools and support) resources you have when facing stressful situations. To illustrate this, you can imagine your reaction when meeting a wild bear being very different depending on whether or not you are a hunter. A hunter will have a better idea of how to handle the situation. In other words, it is not the stress level in itself that determines the reaction; the crucial elements are the ability and tools to influence the situation.

During childbirth, we can translate this into how you experience pain. If you react to the labour pains in a negative way, your body will interpret this as a threatening situation which you do not have the ability to deal with; therefore your body will prepare to run away. If you feel that you know why it hurts, and that you have practical tools to influence your fear, the stress reaction will be reduced and the flight response diminished.

The Birth Without Fear method is based on learning how to *cope* with what is happening, and not trying to take it away or avoid it. This is very much like going for a run. You know from experience that it will be hard and that you are going to have the urge to give up at some points, but you also know from having ran before, that there will be easier parts where you can recover and even enjoy yourself. The most important thing is knowing that it will feel much better once you have finished your run. You have developed a faith in the process and you have worked out strategies to get to the end of the run. You can use the same thought process when it comes to giving birth.

The contractions are like hills when you run; some of them are small, whilst others can feel overwhelming. The pain is the effort that sometimes makes the body ache and throb. As a whole, the experience is like the landscape shifting in colour and form. The reward is the arrival and birth of your baby – this is what makes the experience meaningful!

Coping

1. Comprehensibility

Comprehensibility is an *understanding* of what is happening to you. It means that you are experiencing what happens to you during labour as *orderly, understandable* and *significant*, as opposed to a process which is *chaotic, random* and *inexplicable*. This might involve you gathering knowledge about what happens physically and physiologically during labour. It may also involve you understanding how labour might bring on many contradictory feelings and emotions, and that this is normal. Comprehensibility also entails understanding the specific purpose of pain during labour and how it helps to move the birth process along.

2. Manageability

Manageability implies the trust you have in your own *resources* when it comes to handling and facing whatever comes your way during labour. Your level of *influence* in a given situation also plays an important part here. You cannot *control* the natural process of birth, or the contractions and pain, but you can *influence* how you *handle* the contractions by using internal strategies and the four tools.

3. Meaningfulness

Meaningfulness entails experiencing every situation, including demanding and difficult ones, as *meaningful* and *important* for your growth as a human being. It means finding value in *spending time, engaging in* and applying *energy* into the situation. In the context of childbirth, this translates into the belief that the pain is meaningful, regardless of whether you take pain medication or not, and that the whole experience, including the most difficult parts, are important for you and your development. Therefore, finding *confidence* and *meaning* in childbirth is an important way of preparing emotionally. The purpose of meaningfulness is to protect you from stress and fear.

We are supposed to give birth when we feel safe

Throughout thousands of years of evolution, *oxytocin* has been the hormone the body has chosen as its most important hormone during childbirth to stimulate contractions. Oxytocin is part of our 'peace and calm' system. It is also referred to as the 'love hormone' or the 'feel-good hormone'. The peace and calm system is part of the parasympathetic nervous system, while the stress reaction belongs to the sympathetic nervous system. Together they make up the autonomic nervous system.

Professor Kerstin Uvnäs Moberg has conducted extensive research into this crucial and important hormone. In addition to its function in stimulating contractions during labour, oxytocin also releases a sort of antistress function in the body and is produced when you feel safe, relaxed, calm and good in yourself. Oxytocin is connected to many positive physical and emotional functions such as rest, cell renewal, increasing blood flow to our inner organs, healing muscles and tissue, relationships, feelings of trust, love and pleasure and so much more. Oxytocin also alleviates anxiety and has a pain-relieving quality. The pain is registered, however is not felt so strongly and is not as threatening. It also plays an important role in breastfeeding, bonding with your baby and in the working of contractions.

It is fascinating that the body has chosen oxytocin, which is connected to trust, love and safety, as the key hormone during childbirth. These emotions are not what most people think of connected to birth. The fact that our body, throughout its evolution, has chosen oxytocin as its main hormone for childbirth tells us that we are, in fact, meant to give birth when we feel *safe*. Keeping the evolutionary perspective in mind, giving birth while feeling safe plays an extremely important part for the survival of our species. 'Safety' settles in when we observe our environment and see no signs of threat or danger.

Feeling safe, in turn, tells the body that the chance of survival is high for both the mother and baby; this lets us release the incredible, innate capacity we have to give birth. This positive, physiological spiral is completely *automatic* and is physiologically ready *if* you feel safe and calm. The peace and calm system and the hormone oxytocin can therefore be seen as a 'physiological yes' from the body, since its primary message is safety and reassurance that things are the way they are supposed to be for the mother and the baby.

The four tools you will soon learn more about will help you reduce the negative stress caused by fear, and instead help you to feel safer. In turn the feelings of trust and safety will activate the physiological peace and calm system and the hormone oxytocin. Oxytocin can also be released in response to touch and tenderness, and it induces the feeling of safety, trust, love and calmness and is the primary hormone within relationships. Therefore the book also includes important guidelines for your support person.

Placebo effect

The 'positive placebo effect' is another important component in counteracting fear and stress. We all have this fantastic inherent capability. By *believing* in a *positive* outcome, the body's own system of power and positive energy is stimulated. The body releases substances that help, rather than hinder you.

We know a lot about how negative feelings affect our system, but not much about the effects of positive emotions and how they work. For a long time, science has been looking at what makes us unhealthy and sick, both physically and mentally, but not at what makes us healthy. Emotions like *happiness, joy, awe, self-worth* and *delight* are still relatively unexplored territories. This is about to change, however. Positive psychology, which focuses on what makes us healthy and feel good, is becoming more and more popular. Positive emotions kickstart the reward system in the brain and reduce the release of stress hormones, whilst lowering the heartrate and helping you to relax. This placebo effect has been well known for a long time. It used to be thought of as something negative since doctors would get positive results in clinical trials after having given their patients sugar pills instead of real medicine. Today, we understand that the placebo effect is part of the body's intrinsic ability to self-heal and self-soothe.

I was attending a birth where the woman had previously had a caesarean section. It had been a negative experience for her, and this time she wanted to do things differently. Her mind was set on having a vaginal birth. Her labour started, and the days came and went. Even though it took a long time and there were a few obstacles along the way, she never hesitated or changed her mind. She was completely set on giving birth vaginally, and so she did. However, she had no preconceptions about how long the birth was going to take or what it was going to be like. She was mentally prepared for a second caesarean, but she knew there was also a good chance that things would turn out the way she wanted them to. After her baby was born, she was delighted and felt that her dream had come true. By creating realistic and positive mental images of the birth, you too can access the same inner power.

The reason I write 'realistic' mental images is that unrealistic expectations that do not match your actual abilities can have the opposite effect. If the woman mentioned above had focused on not having an epidural, or demanded that it had to be a quick birth, or that she was going to experience nothing but joy all the time, her reaction afterwards could very well have been the opposite. She could have ended up being sad, disappointed or angry.

Try to avoid 'locking' your mind on achieving a 'perfect birth' or reaching a specific emotional state. Try not to decide in advance how you are going to feel or react, or how the birth will proceed. Instead, be open to the possibility that things may happen in many different ways. Imagine yourself being prepared and able to handle different scenarios. This mind set will help you prepare to handle the unknown.

Exercise: Empowerment

1. Visualise and write down the birth as an open-ended event where you allow for different emotions to take part. The goal of this exercise is to be open minded and present in what happens. Focus inwards rather than outwards. Welcome all emotions and feelings, and picture how you are going to get help and support from the people around you. Practise having the mindset of being kind towards yourself and not demanding too much of yourself.

2. Imagine a staircase of emotional goals. Make the first step easy and realistic. It can be to handle one contraction at a time, or to not tense up during the contraction, or to use the tools to hold fear at bay. The next step might be a little harder. It could be the decision as to whether or not to use pain relief. This may lead to you being able to gain the satisfaction of handling the first step before going on to the next.

Trust

An extremely important emotion which will help you during labour is *trust*. Trust means having confidence in the fact that things will work out fine, and that there is something that provides support regardless of whether or not you have any religious faith. Trust will shelter you from fear, stress and anxiety. You can lean on it in times of weakness and it can be a source of strength. Trust is there as a foundation for when you deal with the uncertain and unpredictable aspects of life. Where there is no trust, negative feelings and thoughts can grow and take over.

People today place great trust in society and the things around them, but not so much when considering their own body. The self-healing aspects of the human body are overlooked and instead we put a lot of faith in medical science. The feeling of being an active participant and being included in the birth disappears if you completely give yourself over to hospital care in the belief that the staff can handle the birth better than you can. Hospitals are partly to blame for this attitude, since many things in their environment, alongside the guidelines surrounding childbirth, signal danger. In order to better be able to access our inner feelings of trust, childbirth needs to be seen, both by the health care professionals and by you, as a *natural and healthy process* rather than primarily posing as a potential risk. We need to remember that birth is the only healthy process we bring into the hospital, only to be prepared for the few times it is medically necessary.

To protect against fear and stress during labour, it is necessary to build a foundation of trust. The ability to have this trust is dependent on your life history, but I believe that this trust is innate and that you can access it within you if you try. There are probably several things in your everyday life that might be risky, but that you still have faith and trust in. You might feel trust every time you sit down in an aeroplane, or start the car, or make an important decision. All these things would be much more difficult if you were tormented by crippling anxiety.

It is not important exactly who, or what, you put your faith or trust in. You might feel trust in your body or in the knowledge it contains. You might put your faith in the hospital and the competence of the staff, in your partner, or your doula, or even your baby. All these factors play an important part when it comes to letting go and allowing your body to give birth. Having faith and trust in your body is an active choice that serves only to empower you.

Exercise: Trust

You can actively stimulate your trust leading up to the birth. You can find it, even if it might be hidden behind life's demands or any negative experiences you might have had. Having trust does not mean having control of the process or of your reactions. Trust reinforces the feeling within you of being an active participant in your life, as opposed to merely being an observer. Therefore, you should write down two or three sentences you can use as affirmations.

Meaningfulness

Meaningfulness and trust are closely related. Both feelings trigger the peace and calm system and the *placebo effect*. Meaningfulness can protect you from negative emotions that can lead to fear. By finding meaning, birth becomes a meaningful event in itself. For example, you can view the pain as meaningful by learning about its function. Meaningfulness can also carry a bigger, more spiritual or existential meaning. Think about what giving birth can mean to you. In what way do you think giving birth can change your relationship with yourself and with your limitations? What does giving birth mean to you, based on who you are? Could the pain have an emotional element? Finding a deeper meaning for giving birth can take time and does not happen overnight. It is important to keep in mind that it is a process that contains several steps.

The meaning of childbirth is as unique and as complex as each individual life. One woman found her meaning when, after twenty-four hours of unsuccessful inductions, she had to say 'stop' and request a caesarean section. By making this decision, she grew as a person and thought of childbirth as an empowering and positive event. Another woman found meaning when she was able to give birth without using pain medication, through the help of her partner, doula and midwife. This was a source of strength for her for many years afterwards. A third woman drew her strength from the fact that she dared to give birth at all, using all the pain relief she could get. After this, she felt she could face other frightening situations in her life. What all these women have in common is that they all decided to face their own fears and not let them take over and control them. All three women demonstrated faith and trust in the meaning of the birth process. You too have the power to create your own unique journey and meaning.

Exercise: Meaning

The following exercises aim to create a feeling of meaning. Write down and discuss the following with your support person:

1. What is the meaning of pain to you? Write down one or two clear sentences.
2. What are your spiritual and existential thoughts about childbirth? What bigger meaning or perspective can giving birth have? In what way do you think giving birth can change you and your limitations and help you to grow? What does giving birth mean to you, personally?

Actively choose

Be active and choose a meaning to access the positive systems in your body. Find your own meaning to giving birth and repeat it over and over. Your meaning can be something grand, but also deeply personal.

Examples:

- 'Giving birth is meaningful to me because I...'
- 'The purpose of pain is it helps my baby be born.'
- 'The purpose of the birth process is for me to develop and grow...'
- 'I understand the function of pain. It...'

Be kind to yourself

Before we go on, I would like to share an important point that I would like you to carry with you. A problem that often arises when talking about childbirth, womanhood, or being responsible for yourself, is that many women feel they must *accomplish* something by giving birth. Then, when they cannot 'live up to the norm', they feel like they have failed. Try, therefore, not to view labour as something that needs to be 'achieved'. I have learnt by experience how difficult it is to know precisely how you are going to react, or what you are going to feel during labour. Do not judge your feelings as being right or wrong. The aim is not about never feeling afraid, and the goal is not to give birth completely without doubt. In other words, you should not be afraid of being afraid! The objective, rather, is to avoid letting fear take root and have a detrimental hold over the process. Look at fear as a natural part of labour and learn how to handle it however it may surface.

Look only to yourself and cultivate love and respect for your inner boundaries and whatever obstacles you encounter. Remember that everyone has their own journey, their own unique experience and their own discoveries. You need to feel that you are supported, respected and that people listen to you, based on who you are. If you do, you will automatically be more forgiving towards yourself and, in addition, you will also feel empowered by knowing you did your best. Your attitude will also become more open minded and you will not compare yourself with others, or feel like you need to be on the defensive when hearing other people's stories. By only comparing with yourself, you will find ways to grow; your eyes will be opened to new options and opportunities which prior you had not realised, or even thought possible.

Respect yourself and your emotions. Think of fear as an internal emotional challenge that you can take charge of. Avoid labelling yourself as 'the scared one' or 'the brave one'. Instead, try to see fear as a natural part of the process and look at labour as an opportunity to grow. Think that you are doing the best that you can, and accept that this is enough, because you are the only one who can determine what is right for you. Focus on what you can handle and view every step you take as a win.

Exercise

Say out loud or think the following every day:
'I will not judge myself.'
'I will be patient and forgiving in the way I treat myself.'
'I will support and love myself in the same way I would support, respect and accept my best friend, my children, or someone else close to me.'

Common concerns before labour

Giving birth and being born are both natural and healthy physiological, emotional and psychological events. Today it often seems to appear that childbirth has been transformed into a medical event, like an operation carried out on the body. However, childbirth is not just a physiological event; you also give birth whilst engaging your emotions and your thoughts. Therefore, it is important to look at childbirth as a complex entity, where your emotions contribute significantly to the medical and physiological event. Understanding the normal birth process and your accompanying emotions, thoughts and fears is, for this reason, an important part of your birth preparation.

Before we move on and look at the normal birth process, I would like to shed some light on a couple of common thoughts and concerns. Fear of giving birth should be seen as *normal*, as it is a natural part of the change process a woman goes through. You will have many questions which you will want answering to help you understand the challenge ahead. Will I be able to handle the birth? Will my body be able to cope? The questions can also be spiritual or existential. What is the purpose of the pain? You might not even know specifically why you are anxious, because the worry is more about facing something unknown and uncertain, or that you have heard it is very painful, ever since you were a child. Many women also feel ashamed at the thought of, for example, defecating during childbirth, or fear that they will not like their pregnant bodies, or that their partner will look at them differently.

To be able to process these thoughts and emotions, you need to be seen, respected and listened to. Your feelings should always be taken seriously, however irrational they might appear to others. You need to accept and respect all emotions, but be mindful and work actively to process them, so that they do not overwhelm you. Science actually tells us that women who *expect* a *negative* birth experience *will* evaluate their childbirth as negative after the birth. It can be a self-fulfilling prophecy, where the negative energies release blocking substances that work against the body. This reaction is called *nocebo*, or the negative expectation effect; it is the opposite of the positive expectation effect, or placebo, we discussed earlier.

You do not have to eradicate fear entirely to prevent this, but you do need to distance yourself from it somewhat. You can accept its existence, but actively choose not to react to it, nor allow it to take over. Decide beforehand to have as a goal to learn to *deal with fear*, rather than trying to eradicate it. It makes sense, therefore, to take a closer look at common sources of fear, so that you get an opportunity to reflect on your worries beforehand. This will help you develop a more realistic and deeper understanding of possible fears.

Two types of fear

After many years of working on the maternity ward, I feel I can distinguish between two different kinds of fear when it comes to childbirth. The first type involves women who have either been close to someone who has had a traumatic birth experience or they themselves have had a first-hand experience of a traumatic birth. It can involve labour and birth complications or of being alone. This fear is always connected to the actual situation.

The second type of fear includes women who have unresolved issues from earlier events in their lives. Women in the first group can be helped by taking specific steps to prevent the trauma from recurring. The second group can partly be helped by this approach, but it is usually not enough. They need assistance in gaining an understanding of the underlying cause of their fear.

I was hired to be a doula for a woman who had a very bad relationship with her mother. Her mother was a drug addict and had not been able to give her daughter any basic sense of security. The woman and her partner hired me because of her fear of birth. We worked on this fear a lot throughout her pregnancy. During one of our talks, I asked if she had any fears about becoming a mother. She reflected on this and realised she was afraid to birth her baby. What if she could not love a child? What if she were to harm her baby emotionally, just like she had been harmed? She was given the space to articulate her thoughts and throughout the conversation she could see how she already was a good mother by daring to talk about these issues and being aware of them. She felt hope returning and was then looking forward to meeting her baby. This made her fear of delivery more or less vanish. One month later, she gave birth to a son and the birth went well.

It is not necessary to go through extensive therapy to be able to handle fear. The simple act of trying to look at the problem from several different angles can help you articulate the fears and overcome any emotional hurdles you might be carrying with you. This process can transform the difficult aspects of life into strengths.

A previous negative birth experience

The fear that occurs after a previous negative birth experience is often connected to an underlying distrust, either of the healthcare system, of one's partner or of one's own body. Usually the fear itself is concretely connected to the previous experience. You might have had preconceived expectations about what the birth would be like. When the labour did not happen as you thought it would, you might have felt disappointed. Another scenario is that you might have looked forward to the birth, without any fear whatsoever, only to discover that it was not at all what you had expected; the force and pain might have been stronger and harder to handle than you had imagined. Alternatively, the worst thing might not have been the pain, but was the feelings of being alone and vulnerable.

To be able to process the previous experience you need to be allowed to talk about it. The thankfulness you feel about the fact that everything went well from a medical point of view might stand in direct conflict with your emotional experience, where everything definitely did not go well. You might think it is taboo to discuss your feelings, or you might not even be aware of an inner turmoil. Copious amounts of energy are wasted and, most importantly, the event is not being discussed and processed emotionally. Sometimes you do not know who is to blame, but you are just left with a feeling that you needed something more, something that the healthcare system could not offer.

Try to view the previous experience as meaningful, as it will help you understand how you can prepare for the upcoming birth. *It is possible* to heal the wounds from past experiences with the help of a new birth, and I have been fortunate to witness this amazing transformation many times. Memories of the new experience cover the old wounds and replace them with new, positive emotions.

Negative influences from others

Fear can come both from within ourselves and from outside of us. Some people have an almost pathological need to tell horrific birth stories as soon as they spot a pregnant woman. It is not okay to do so! You have the right to put your foot down and tell them to stop. To protect yourself you need to kindly, but firmly, indicate that you do not want to hear what the person wants to tell you, at least till after you have given birth. Instead, try talking to people who will bring out the positive, empowering images of birth. Aim to cut out any negative influences as much as possible.

Too much information about what can go wrong during pregnancy and delivery can also create anxiety and fear. Ask yourself if it really is necessary to know everything that could possibly go wrong, or whether it might be better to trust that you will get all the help possible *if* something happens. It can be difficult to handle the knowledge that something might go wrong, but this knowledge is an inexorable part of life as a whole. For example, when you get in your car you do not automatically think of the possible accidents you might get into or of all the horrible injuries those accidents might involve.

I am aware that these things are not directly comparable. However, it can help to put things into perspective if you think about how impossible it would be to drive if you were to focus on all the things that could go wrong. I do not suggest you should repress your feelings about birth, but it might be better to talk about what you are afraid of. You will then have the opportunity to find out if other people share your worries, as well as help you to understand where the fear originates from.

Support

Support and security have an enormous influence on negative emotions and stress reactions and many women realise they will need a lot of support during childbirth. Therefore, it is important to feel seen and respected and not to be alone while giving birth. This includes when you use pain relief since women using pain relief are more easily left alone without support.

Take your emotions seriously. Talk to your partner about what is important to you. Ask him or her to be honest about their feelings. This is a new situation for both of you and if your partner is as insecure as you are, it can be a good idea to look for alternatives. Maybe you can get the help of a doula, a friend, or a mother. Women's views of their relationship to their partner can improve when an extra support person is present during labour. If you feel you did not get enough support from your partner, you might feel hurt and deserted, and it can take a long time to rebuild that trust. However, if your partner can share the responsibility with someone else, the extra support can actually help strengthen your partner in their role as support person. You should also let the maternity ward staff know what sort of assistance you feel that you need. You might want them to praise you, be close to you, to use certain words or to do something entirely different. Many women do not do this, because they do not want to be in the way, or seen as bothersome. Since the staff do not know you personally, however, it is very valuable for them to be given this kind of direction.

Your support person also needs information about how they can assist you in better ways. The support person is often expected to automatically know how to support a woman during labour, even though daily life is very different from childbirth. It is therefore unfair to expect the support person to know what you need in this situation. There is a chapter dedicated specifically to the support person at the end of this book.

Exercise: Reduce the fear of not receiving adequate support

- Talk about what kind of support both of you need.
- Be honest.
- Let the staff know in what ways you want to be helped.

Complications

Fear of something happening to you or your baby is a natural survival instinct that is set in motion when you become pregnant. This can be seen as preparation for parenthood and the responsibilities that come with it. Allow yourself to talk about these feelings, your doubts and your hopes with a midwife, your partner or a close friend. It can be worth keeping in mind that the entire healthcare system is based on a 'just in case' principal. This means that many precautions are taken despite there being no real danger. Complications are rare, and babies have amazing physiology and reserves for labour and birth. However, if a complication arises you need to trust in the staff and have faith in their competence.

Sometimes, things happen that we do not want to happen, and you need to consider that thought as well; this fear can end up taking up too much space though. Ask yourself why you do not feel you can trust yourself and your baby. In which situations in life have you had to carry a lot of doubt or sorrow? Find the courage to bring this forward so that you can get help processing these feelings. Could it be that you guard yourself from feeling disappointed in life? Can you find something that can help you endure what you cannot control? Perhaps this will allow you to build new trust, even if the old emotions still linger.

Exercise: Reduce the fear of complications

- Think about what you need in order to strengthen yourself. Look for positive role models and stories that can help you, then actively bring them forward.
- Think about your worry as a natural way of preparing for motherhood. You might have to wade through your worst thoughts and fears. Once you say them out loud, their power wains and you feel less afraid.
- Ask the maternity ward staff about anything specific you want to know or get information about.

Medical interventions

It is common for women to have a fear of medical interventions, such as caesarean sections, vacuum extractions or injections/infusions. This can also be seen as connected to loss of control, since you no longer are in charge, which can therefore make you feel unsafe.

In order to process these thoughts and feelings try to pinpoint what it is you find uncomfortable or worrying. Consider reading up on what happens during the medical intervention you are specifically afraid of so that you gain more information and understanding. In extreme cases cognitive therapy can be useful in helping you deal with your particular fear. If you are having a planned caesarean section and you are feeling very anxious you could possibly contact the Labour Ward Manager and ask if you are able to see the operating theatre and discuss your care. This will strengthen your sense of being in control and will help you find coping strategies that work for you.

These obvious, real fears can also conceal a more subtle fear which is connected to your sense of self and lack of trust. Try to express in words the feeling connected to the specific situation. Remember that the staff are experts at what they do and are there to do everything they can to help you. Tell your partner or support person how you want them to help you emotionally; perhaps you want them to remind you that everything is as it should be, and that they should repeat this to you again and again.

Exercise: Reduce the fear of medical interventions

- Are you afraid of losing control? Are there positive and negative ways of losing control? Learn the tools and use them in these situations.
- Are you afraid of signs that something is wrong?
- Are you afraid of doubting yourself when it comes to dealing with whatever happens?

Losing control

Letting go and *allowing* the natural birth process to happen is very important. This can, at the same time, also be very scary, and many women get trapped in trying to control the process. Many women fear losing control when giving birth. Losing control can, of course, be frightening, especially if it is connected to stress and fear. Giving birth can also involve you losing control over your body to some extent. For some women, this stands in stark contrast to their everyday lives.

There is, however, both positive and negative control. Trusting your body, feeling participatory in the decisions being made and having the tools necessary to follow the process are examples of *positive control*. Feeling in command of the things you can influence or steer is the foundation of positive control. You cannot control the birth process, but you can however actively work with handling the fear and the contractions. *Negative control* is trying to control what is *outside of your influence*, such as pain, the physical birth process or any necessary bodily functions.

You can also ask yourself whether or not the loss of control is always a negative thing. *Letting go* of control, as opposed to *losing* control, can be a good thing. The techniques described in this book will show you how to relinquish control and allow the birth to progress. Letting go and surrendering are closely related. A sense of trust and security is essential to be able to surrender to something. Therefore, a good way to prepare might be to think about what circumstances will allow you to surrender to a bodily experience. What should your surroundings be like for you to do this?

Exercise: Reduce the fear of losing control

- Define what 'losing control' means to you.
- Describe the help you would like to receive if you get stuck in these emotions.
- Articulate ways in which 'letting go' of control could be positive for you.

Exercise: Letting go of control – surrendering

This simple exercise will help you practise surrendering and letting go of control and it aims to train your body to relax your muscles. You use the body's movements to 'unlock' a mental block. You can use this exercise during labour, but also in other situations when you feel mentally frustrated.

1. Stand up straight.
2. Notice if your body feels in balance or if you need to adjust something.
3. Lift your arms so that they point straight out from your body.
4. When exhaling, lower your arms slowly and let your head fall slightly back while you bend your knees gently.
5. Repeat this a couple of times.
6. It is common for your exhalation to become audible when you perform the movement.

Pain

Thinking about the pain of childbirth, especially if you are a first-time mother, can mean you are facing the unfamiliar and unknown. You may question whether you will be able to handle it and wonder if you will feel scared of the pain, process and intensity. This is not unusual, and is in fact a normal feeling, since the contractions during childbirth can be one of the strongest sensations of pain a woman will experience. However, this does not automatically mean that the pain during labour is destructive or negative.

What we need to learn is that we are capable of handling the pain and *how* to do it. This includes if you use pain relief or have caesarean section. Pain relief does not replace the need for support and you will still need to cope with some level of emotional and physical challenges and pain in birth.

Pain during normal labour can be described as constructive pain (the body is working as it should) and is very different from pain caused by an injury or trauma. Destructive pain signals injury, while pain during labour is a sign of the physical transformations happening in your body. We also know that it is coming and that it is part of something healthy and natural. It can of course be intense and very challenging, but it is still not a sign of something bad happening. On the contrary, it is part of something positive and purposeful – the birth of your baby. Pain caused by an injury does not come and go, but instead tends to persist. Normal labour pain always offers breaks in between contractions when you can rest and recoup your energy.

The claim that pain always functions as a warning signal is therefore not true. Pain can many times be linked to organic functions, signalling a forthcoming event, for example with ovulatory pain. It can also be naturally experienced as the growing pains felt by a child, the pain of a tooth pushing through the gums in an infant, or the cramps felt when the egg and lining of the womb are shed during menstruation. These pains all have a valid reason for their existence.

It is the way you *relate* to the pain on an *emotional* level that determines if it is perceived as *positive or negative*. Pain alone is not usually what women experience as negative during labour. Instead, what is traumatic is generally the negative emotions connected to the pain. They might feel alone, scared or trapped. These feelings give way to suffering and distress. It is possible, however, to experience pain without suffering, and indeed to suffer but without actually being in pain, like emotional pain. If you have a solid base of inner trust, a support system surrounding you and the means to handle whatever comes your way, the pain does not have to involve suffering. The pain can be limited to a strong and powerful sensation that you simply work your way through and cope with.

Therefore you can influence *how* you experience pain during labour. Pain is experienced differently and is less threatening if you feel secure, safe and calm. This is because in this state your body is able to produce oxytocin, which has pain reducing qualities and dampens anxiety. Many of the women who have given birth using the Birth Without Fear method describe this difference; they experienced the pain of the contractions very differently when they felt supported, secure and had the necessary tools to handle the situation, even when it became more challenging and more intense.

Acceptance

Acceptance can be a useful tool to help you handle pain. There are
times when it is a positive thing to accept what we *cannot change*,
and not try to change it, escape or run from it. In order to paint a
picture of what this can entail, I want to give an example from a
birth I was involved in.

At the time, I was working as an assistant nurse. The midwife
told me the woman was of another country and language and was
struggling quite a bit. She complained constantly and had difficulty
walking or even moving to the bathroom. When I got into the
room she was lying on the bed with her eyes closed, complaining
verbally, her body completely limp. The staff had become more and
more frustrated with her, since it was hard to communicate and

help her properly. I had heard that this behaviour was common among women from this part of Europe.

I grew more and more fascinated by her actions. Her voice turned into a deep lamentation during each contraction, her movements became slow and introverted, but what really struck me was that she was not going anywhere. In order to get her to move to the toilet, you had to basically carry her. Her body showed no signs of stress or wanting to run away.

Hours went by, and the birth process moved forward slowly. She moaned her way through the contractions in her own way, calmly and deeply. At one point, the midwife thought that she might need pain medication after all and asked if she wanted any. The woman lifted her blurry eyes and looked at her as if she had not quite understood the question, after which she declined resolutely. She fell asleep occasionally, and her husband always remained at her side, without intervening or trying to change anything.

At no time did I notice any fear or stress in her; she had accepted her situation and the pain completely. She did not try to run away from it or get around it. She had understood and accepted that everything that was happening was inevitable, and from this, she found the energy to keep going, despite her moaning and complaining. As soon as her baby was born, her behaviour changed entirely and she lovingly greeted her baby, her face beaming with pride and happiness.

Exercise: Acceptance

You can use these exercises during contractions, or at any time during labour. They also work when you find yourself in a stressful situation, or if you experience feelings you find difficult to handle. You can also use them when you are in pain, are feeling bad or when you simply want to access positive energy. This first exercise is extremely useful when the pain is building up and you sense that you are starting to tense up.

Choose to Accept;

1. Sit comfortably.
2. Decide to be accepting.
3. Accept with your heart, your brain and your body – accept with your entire being.
4. Put your acceptance into words and say them out loud or quietly to yourself, *'It is okay. This moment is okay. I allow it even if I do not like it or want it, and even if I wish it was different, I let it come, and I let it go.'*
5. *' I accept the pain and let it come.'*

Breathing;

1. Sit down uncomfortably, and yes, I mean *uncomfortably.*
2. Take a deep, soft breath that feels good to you. Notice how your ribcage expands.
3. Then, let the air flow out while you let your body relax.

4. Turn the palms of your hands up and open them. Take a couple of breaths at your own pace. Feel how your open hands help you to receive, accept and allows the signals your body sends out to flow. This is more difficult to do with clenched fists.

Tearing

It comes as no surprise that many women fear tearing. However, it is almost as if we have taught ourselves to think in a negative and terrifying way. The pelvic floor, perineum, labia and vagina are designed to be able to adjust themselves to accommodate the baby's journey. This accommodation sometimes results in a natural laceration. The shape of the vagina and the tissues surrounding it are made to be able to tear a little to make the passing of the baby smoother, and to heal quickly afterwards. It is nothing major, and many women often *do not* even notice a laceration occurring during birth. Of course, you might feel sore after the birth, but this is normal whether you have had a laceration or not. We need to erase the old, negative way of looking at this and instead actively embrace a new way of seeing it as something normal.

In order to avoid more severe lacerations, you need support and help during the pushing phase so that you do not get caught up in fear and stress, rather let the pushing take its time. There are many different opinions on the best way to avoid tearing while pushing the baby out. People discuss whether the midwife should support the perineum, or if other medical measures should be taken. These issues are important, but I think the most important thing is for the woman to get help in handling her fear. Fear will affect the elasticity of the muscles and tissues in a negative way. A pelvic floor that resists and tightens is not ready to let a baby through. Fear will tense and tighten the muscles, causing the birth process to stall in order for you to move to someplace safe.

If the mother has a sense of trust and the atmosphere around her is supportive and calm, the blood circulation to the muscles and tissues will increase, the muscles can relax and soften, and the baby will be able to pass through more easily. To encourage these emotions, you need to be in a calm, safe and unforced environment. Listen to the instructions of the midwife and, if all is well with you and baby, let them know you want to take your time.

Exercise

Exercise: Preparations for the pushing phase

- Shift your perspective and look at a small laceration as a natural part of giving birth.
- Prevent larger tears by allowing yourself to take time, by not letting fear take over and by making sure you feel safe.
- Understand how your body is constructed. Build faith around the fact that your body is made to be able to handle all parts of childbirth.

Elin's Birth Story

After delivering my first baby, I did not feel well at all. I had a great need to process everything, but the feeling of disappointment would not loosen its grip. I had been so prepared, energised and rested, and I had a high threshold for pain. Despite this, I ended up with medical procedures, an episiotomy, a vacuum extraction birth and a deep concern for the baby.

Immediately afterwards, I was in pain from the stitches and I had a hard time bonding with my baby. All I could think about was the 36-hour-long birth process and everything that had happened.

Before the second birth, I tried not to make the same mistake of connecting my self-esteem to the birth process. I knew, however, that I needed a positive birth experience to have the energy necessary to handle a new-born baby and a three-year-old. I contacted a doula to increase my chances of having the kind of birth I wanted and to feel like I had done what I could. It was a relief to have someone beside me who knew what I wanted and who could support me when things got difficult. Just as the time before, I preferred not to have any medical pain relief – perhaps just gas and air. I just wanted to know how much pain nature intended me to feel and I wanted to do everything in my power to avoid complications for my baby. I was given an injection during my first labour, on the assumption that I was too tired and to help me when receiving contraction stimulation medicine. I am not sure if this was the right decision and I wonder if the stress I felt from the beginning of labour effected my baby.

My overriding concern this time was that I would get depressed after yet another disappointing birth. I was also worried I would be taken by surprise by the pain, since I had hardly experienced any pain last time. I spoke to my doula about my experiences and I felt I got a little further processing things. I had found women who understood how I had felt cheated by my experience and how I no longer trusted my body the way I used to. I decided this time I needed not to 'run away', but instead to relax and let go.

After two false alarms with practice contractions, I was happy when it seemed like labour had started for real – and on the due date as well. The contractions came quickly and we were admitted at 10.35 pm on a Sunday night. At the hospital everything changed and it felt scary and uncomfortable. I no longer wanted to give birth and I wished I could just take a pill to stop the process. The examination showed I was only three centimetres dilated and the membranes were intact. This left me with a heavy feeling. Perhaps my body could not do this after all? My baby's head was also facing the wrong way, just like last time. This was not a good start and all the old feelings returned. I hesitated to call my doula. I thought I could not ask her to be at the hospital for 20 hours straight and it would be better to save her for when a real crisis happened. I ended up calling her in after all, since I felt scared and vulnerable at the hospital. With my partner, I managed to walk a few turns in the hospital hallway before she showed up. The contractions came frequently, and it felt good having my doula and my partner taking it in turns to massage me.

During the contractions, I worked consciously to not trigger the fight-or-flight response. I fought hard to keep my feet firmly on the ground and my face relaxed. It was impossible to keep my shoulders and back relaxed though. My support people helped me with this by giving me a massage. I managed to stay away from any feelings of panic and the contractions kept coming. I was happy the contractions came as closely and regularly as they did; this meant the staff would not send me home at least. I had no other pain relief in mind, other than my TENS-machine that was running at half speed. I did not even consider using gas and air. Had a midwife suggested it, I would probably have lost my confidence, which might have made me more aware of the difficulties. Besides, I thought I would struggle throughout the whole night, so it was best to hold fire. It was somewhat frightening how hard it already was though. Would I not be able to get through it without painkillers if it went on for too long? It was not exactly painful, but rather a scary sense of pressure bearing down on me. 'Do not be scared,' I kept repeating to myself. 'It is just an uncomfortable sensation. It is part of the process.' Time went by quickly, and two hours passed in a flash.

At 1.15 am, the midwife thought I looked a little sweaty and wanted to see how things had been moving along. I felt so happy when she said I was dilated a full ten centimetres and the baby was on its way! No wonder I had felt pressure. I had a lot of strength left and I dared to give birth. After making sure it was okay, I pushed with each contraction and after three, my baby son was born.

Two tiny stitches were required but they really didn't hurt. My legs shook violently, but it was mostly just comical. I did not want to sleep. I was savouring my birth experience and treated myself to a couple of paracetamols for the after-pains. Importantly, I got a completely fresh start when I became a mother of two.

One of my first thoughts right afterwards was how unbelievably strong I had been during my first birth, which had been so much harder. Why had I felt like a failure, when, in fact, it had been a great achievement? Before my second birth, I had accepted that I would have to live the rest of my life with these feelings of failure. Now, I am grateful for the humbleness I have experienced. The most important support this time came from my doula, who always shared her belief in my body and its ability to give birth. When I let go of my doubts, I dared to stay in the moment and give birth in my own way.

The birth

You now have the knowledge of how stress and fear can affect a woman's body and mind. You have more tools and strategies to face and handle the positive as well as the negative emotions that might emerge during labour. Now we will look at the natural and healthy birth process and how your body is made for the physical changes that will occur, so that you can differentiate between this natural process and the most common reactions to fear.

Pain connected to labour often *triggers* fear, which in turn triggers involuntary stress reactions. This commonly happens as a result of you not understanding the purpose of the pain, which then therefore only feels destructive and meaningless. The pain is, in this case, nothing but an unpleasant sensation that keeps growing and growing.

After an energetic workout you might experience muscle pain. It can be quite sore at times, but it never frightens you because you recognise it as a sign that your body has worked hard and is becoming stronger. If that same sensation were to hit you suddenly while you were relaxing on the couch, it might frighten you since you would not know where it came from.

Therefore, in order to avoid becoming scared, you need to understand that the pain is a messenger which serves to update you on the physical changes happening during labour. This knowledge will challenge the perception of pain as an external force that takes over your body and that you cannot control. By understanding contractions and their function, you create meaningful, mental images, which make the contractions more comprehensible and concrete. Childbirth is then no longer a threat, but rather a physically demanding job for which you have all the necessary tools at your disposal.

There is, of course, a possibility that you will experience minimal pain giving birth and that through support, security and love, will manage to transform the physical labour into a different kind of sensation. These women may experience the contractions as a kind of force or intense sensation. However, for the majority of women some level of pain is usually associated with this important work, even with pain medication on board. Therefore, saying that there is no pain associated with childbirth is for most women not true. What we can say, is that childbirth is entirely normal, and that the body is fully equipped to handle this process.

The perfect body

I have written this book with normal and healthy childbirth in mind. If you have any specific worries or concerns, it would of course be advisable to explore those in greater detail. My view is that if something unexpected or out of the ordinary occurs during labour, the staff will let you know what is happening, what they are going to do about it and why. Today, births taking place in hospitals, as well as at home, are safe thanks to the extensive knowledge and skills of the midwives and other healthcare personnel, both in how to foresee and in preventing possible complications.

We should not forget however that the body is a marvellous creation, where hundreds of thousands of physiological functions interplay seamlessly every day. All these functions are physiologically automatic, as is the birth physiology. Your body knows how to do it and your most important job is to have the least amount of resistance to this hard, but very important work the body needs to do in order to birth your baby.

Your body

Before we continue, I would like us to take a moment and explore the different parts of your birthing body, as well as go through a couple of important terms associated with labour. This section will give you a sense of how amazing your body is and of how everything is structured, interconnected and prepared.

The main anatomy involved in childbirth:

- **Uterus**
- **Cervix**
- **Birth canal/vagina**
- **Opening of the vulva**

The uterus, or 'womb', is a pear-shaped muscle, within which there is a cavity where the baby grows during pregnancy. The uterus of a non-pregnant woman is about the size of a pear and is hidden behind the pubic bone, within the pelvis. During pregnancy it grows simultaneously with the growing baby. Towards the end of the pregnancy it has expanded in size – from level with your pubic bone, up to your ribcage, and at this point it becomes the largest muscle in your body.

The cervix, or 'neck of the womb', connects the uterus to the birth canal. At the beginning of labour, the cervix is around two to three centimetres in length, firm and closed. As labour progresses it shortens ('effaces'), softens and moves forward towards the front of the pelvis. With contractions this ring-shaped cervix gradually widens and opens, until it reaches ten centimetres in diameter and is fully open.

The mucus plug sits in the neck of the cervix during pregnancy and protects the entrance to the uterus. This is the 'show' that is passed vaginally when the cervix begins to soften and shorten in preparation for labour.

The Birth Canal is the vagina, which is a folded passageway connecting the uterus to the opening of the vagina. It is a mucus membrane, able to unfold and expand to let the baby through, then tighten again, a bit like the musical instrument, the accordion.

The outer female vulva consists of two inner labia/lips, then two outer labia. Their vertical shape allows them to fit around the baby's head as it pushes through.

The pelvic floor is the muscular base of the abdomen and is attached to the pelvis. The muscles form a figure-of-eight shape around the urethra at the front, from where you pass urine, the vaginal opening, and the anus – the back passage. It supports and holds up the internal organs of the bladder, uterus and bowels above. These are the muscles you feel if you squeeze around your anus, vagina and urethra.

The perineum is the area of tissue between the anus and the vagina.

The placenta is a temporary organ created specifically for the pregnancy. It is implanted in the uterine lining and connects to the baby via the umbilical cord. The placenta receives oxygen and nutrition from you and transfers these to the baby. Waste products from the baby are also filtered and removed via the placenta. It is a unique organ which belongs to the baby so that they grow and thrive.

Two **membranes** surround the baby and the placenta, providing a sterile sac for the baby to grow inside. Within the sac, the baby is supported and moves around in amniotic fluid. This fluid contains salt, proteins, fats, sugars, hormones and enzymes', but about ninety-five percent of the fluid is simply water. By the end of the last trimester, the amniotic fluid is replaced about every three hours. The sac of amniotic fluid can break just before labour begins or at any time during labour. Occasionally the baby is born with the amniotic sac intact.

The heart of birth

The main part in birth is the work of the uterus and the contractions. The contractions are what moves the process along, whatever phase that labour happens to be in. The word 'contraction' is used as an overall term to describe the enormous muscular work done by the uterus during all phases of labour.

The contraction can be compared to an ocean wave, where all the muscle fibres of the uterus tighten and relax, *over approximately sixty seconds*. The contraction begins, builds up in its intensity, until it reaches its bottom, then subsides, and after these sixty seconds there is a natural pause. Within the contraction itself there is a 'wave' of force; beginning as mild, growing in intensity to its bottom, then subsiding till the womb is at rest.

The direction of the uterus and the baby in the body is down. Therefore it is helpful to imagine the contraction going downwards, and having a bottom, and not a top. When you visualise the contraction, think of it as a wave, like a 'U' shape, rather than as a peak – which is how contractions are usually described and how they appear on a visual display graph of contractions. It is much more strenuous to climb to the top of a mountain than it is to slide passively to the bottom of a wave!

The uterus is made up of smooth muscle fibres. These smooth muscles are not controlled by your will, but are influenced by hormones and feelings, and work automatically. There is another muscle in your body that works in a similar way, the heart. The heart is made of a unique and different kind of muscle, however there are some similarities. The heart muscle also cannot be controlled by our will and works rhythmically, when the atria then ventricles contract, and a relaxation part when the chambers refill with blood.

This intrinsic rhythm is our life force, keeping us alive. Therefore, I like to think of the uterus as the 'heart' of childbirth. The contractions are the heartbeats, the work that the body needs to do that symbolise a movement that pushes the baby closer and closer to you.

The rhythm of contractions

As the heart the uterus has a rhythm during birth; the working part when it contracts, gradually opening the cervix and pushing the baby down, followed by a resting part, when the uterus relaxes, allowing the placenta and baby to be fully oxygenated and the labouring woman to rest. This rhythm, where each contraction has a certain length, followed by a pause, is the key element of birth and your handling focus regardless of which stage you are in. This rhythm is not unusual to your body; rather, it has similarities to your breathing pattern, the way that your muscles can tighten/flex and then relax/extend and other physical patterns like your heart as I already mentioned above.

Nature has designed this rhythm of contractions to be as close to perfection as possible. Labour does not consist of one long contraction or continuous pain, which would result in you becoming exhausted, both mentally and physically. Instead, contractions are divided up into intervals. Hence, an active contraction lasting for approximately sixty seconds is *always* followed by a break or pause.

The length of the contractions varies depending on which stage of the birthing process you are in. During the early stages of labour the contractions might last anywhere from fifteen to sixty seconds and can be irregular in their frequency and duration. When the birth process is more *established*, the contractions become stronger and they tend to be more regular in their frequency, lasting around sixty seconds. Pain during labour is therefore *limited* and surfaces predominately *during contractions* that last about sixty seconds. It is therefore possible to prepare for, and each contraction has a beginning, a middle and an end. It is not endless or constant.

In the early stages of labour the breaks after a contraction could last for half an hour up to several hours. The rest between contractions gets shorter and shorter the closer to actual birth you get. The rests will get shorter, however, the contractions will not get longer.

This built-in rhythm and direction are prerequisites for you to make it through the whole process and provide the power to birth your baby. However, if stress hormone levels are high during labour, you could lose the connection with this rhythm. When this happens, you might *experience* the contractions as a *constant* contraction, and not truly experience or benefit from the rest period in between.

The four tools in this book, and especially the strategy to sigh deeply after each contraction which you will learn more about in the next chapter, will help you to follow this rhythm and work with your body. This will reduce your stress hormone levels, enabling you to maximise breaks between the contractions in order to rest and gather strength. This is important since many women describe lack of sleep as a major obstacle. By making good use of the breaks, you will be able to flow with your body's birthing rhythm, no matter how long labour lasts.

The different stages of labour:

The beginning of labour

Many women wonder how to recognise the beginning of labour.
No two births begin in the same way. I know that this might be
very frustrating to hear for the first-time mother who wants clear
information, but this is also what makes the whole birth process so
special. Every single childbirth brings its own unique variation of
experiences.

Labour might start with:

- An ache similar to menstrual pains. This can be felt
  in the thighs, lower abdomen and/or back.

- The release of the mucus plug. It can look like jelly,
  sometimes stained with blood, or it can be more
  like a lump of mucus. If there are more than a few
  drops of blood and/or a *constant* pain you should
  call a midwife or the hospital and consult with
  them. The mucus plug is sometimes released a week
  or two before the birth, so a released mucus plug
  does not automatically mean you are in labour.
  However, it does show that your body is preparing
  for labour

- The breaking of the amniotic sac – 'waters breaking'. This might happen as an obvious 'pop' with a significant amount of fluid coming out, or it can be a slow trickle. The water can be clear, or it can have a slightly pinkish hue. You should contact the midwife or hospital if you think that your waters have broken. It is especially important to do so if the water leaking is green in colour.

- The beginning of contractions. Commonly they are fairly brief and not very strong in the beginning. The labour could, however, start off with longer and stronger contractions right from the start.

All these things might occur. The signals might be haphazard in the beginning. It is important to remember to let the process take place in its own time. Do not get stressed or frustrated if you cannot read all the signs, or if you feel you do not understand exactly what is happening. Let the birth start peacefully. Try to remain in the moment and take things as they unfold and do not be hard on yourself. It is not a sign of failure if you mistake the signals and you are not as dilated as you had hoped.

Early labour
Early labour is the first phase of labour. The body prepares for the coming birth by fine-tuning all the necessary functions. This phase is like a message from the body telling you how you will have to start working together soon.

The work of the uterus

During this stage of labour, the cervix feels firm, somewhat like the tip of your nose when you touch it with your finger. The first thing that happens during contractions is that the cervix becomes thinner, softer and its opening (the 'cervical os') moves from facing towards the back of your pelvis, to a central position, and then further forward, directed towards the vagina. The cervical opening then continues to widen to about four to five centimetres.

Early labour can last anywhere from a few hours, to a few days. The contractions are usually irregular and the breaks in between them vary in duration. Or, they can be regular for a while, and then stop. During the beginning of labour, the contractions tend to be milder in strength and last anywhere between fifteen to sixty seconds. The breaks can last anywhere between a few minutes to a few hours.

Emotions during early labour

You might be completely unaware of this phase happening at all, or it can feel quite obvious to you. The sensation of the tightenings or contractions at this point can be mild and feel like an ache in the pelvic floor or lower abdomen. This ache will later transform into a more painful sensation in the same region. However, for some women the sensation can be quite strong even during this early stage.

A variety of emotions might surface during the early labour phase. Many women feel happy, excited and filled with expectation as they feel the first contractions and look forward to meeting their baby. This is, however, a time when a lot of women wear themselves out by mentally focusing all their energy on the upcoming birth. It is important to *preserve energy*, not to spend it focusing on every contraction, wondering how long it is going to take, monitoring how long the breaks are. You might also feel confused or frustrated. Has it started for real, or not?

Think of it as a secret that only you know and that is slowly unravelling in your body. Every now and then, you can register the rhythm of the contractions, but you should spend the time in between focusing on other things. Try to distract yourself as much as possible. One couple I was assisting loved to go and look at houses that were for sale, and actually spent the first part of labour viewing properties while the contractions came and went. When they returned home, they relaxed in front of the television. As labour finally intensified, the woman felt she had a lot of mental strength left and she ended up giving birth that same night.

If the pain is intense you might feel scared and if early labour phase goes on for a long time, you might become exhausted. You might go through times when you distrust your body or worry about its ability to handle childbirth – especially if you see little or no progress. However, you can also feel empowered by your ability to let your body do its preparatory work for labour, alongside resting and being ready mentally and physically for the ongoing process. Al of these emotions are normal.

Active labour

Active or established labour is when the cervix goes from approximately five centimetres dilated to ten centimetres or 'fully' dilated. The contractions now have more or less the same duration of about sixty seconds and the breaks between have a regular and steady rhythm. The closer you are to giving birth, the shorter the breaks between contractions become, to the point where the breaks between contractions are lasting about the same length as the contractions themselves. The contractions also become more intense for each centimetre you are dilated, but not longer. You might sometimes experience very strong contractions and still not see any visual results. Remember that your body is working hard in each and every contraction to bring you closer to the goal, even if results are not yet visible.

The work of the uterus

Numerous pain receptors are situated around the cervical opening. This is the way the body is designed, and it works because it is via this information that you constantly are reminded of the progress of labour. Think of the opening of the cervix rather like trying to put a polo-neck sweater over a baby's head. The force of the contractions pulls the sweater over the baby's head little by little. As it can be difficult to understand what causes the pain, picturing the cervix like a rubber band, gradually widening with each contraction can be a helpful visualisation. This can help you understand the purpose of the pain and assist you to realise that it is not there to cause you any harm. *It is the body working as it is designed to.*

At the end of the opening phase, the cervix is ten centimetres dilated and the baby's head is sitting at the top of the birth canal and the vagina, ready to start its journey down, and out into the world. As your baby's head becomes lower in the birth canal the contractions will begin to change in character. At first it may be similar to the feeling that you need to open your bowels, as you feel the pressure of your baby's head bearing down with the contractions. The feeling of an intense pressure with the contractions will take over more and more.

This stage generally lasts a couple of hours up to around one day.

Emotions during active labour

Some women experience the opening phase as chaotic and hard to comprehend. The problem is that this phase is not always clear and distinct. It is not possible to see or feel what the uterus and cervix are doing. Some women, in contrast, find this phase very easy to deal with as there is no requirement to do anything. The woman simply has to let go, whereas the pushing phase that follows usually requires effort.

The most important thing in the opening phase is experiencing the immediate *now*. Focusing on the contraction you are feeling *right now*, or the break you are in *right now* is key. If you start pondering on the number of contractions you might have left, or how long it is going to take, it is as if you are dealing with all the contractions at once. Notions of time only make the process unmanageable. It is important that everyone around you helps to keep the focus on what is behind you, not what is in front of you. The thought of being in pain for another two hours can be unbearable, but if you shift your perspective and deal just with the present, you will be able to handle a lot more than you can imagine. Be mindful and remind yourself to collect your thoughts throughout the process.

During the opening phase you might still feel confused and even wonder whether the labour has started or not. You might, however, feel a sense of empowerment from being able to handle the contractions. It is also common for first-time mothers, who have no previous experience to compare with, to believe that the labour process has progressed further than it actually has at this point.

When the labour starts to accelerate, you might temporarily react with despair or fear, however, you need to adjust to the increased sensation of pain. Do not give up. Simply allow time to pass; if you do this, you will regain confidence and feel secure again. If the labour up until this point has been more drawn out than you expected, it might feel like a heavy burden to think about how difficult the process is and how much still lies ahead. It is common to go back and forth between positive and negative emotions.

When is it time to go?

It is difficult to pinpoint the exact moment when it is time to go to the hospital or birthing centre. Many first-time mothers go too early since they do not have any previous experiences to go by. Understand that this may happen to you as well. However, the four tools can make it feel easier to stay at home a little longer.

Knowing when to go to the hospital can be difficult to judge, even for experienced mothers, since the body might not follow the same pattern as during previous births. There are, however, general guidelines for when it can be time to go. You will need to *call* the maternity unit at the hospital where you are birthing your baby, or the midwife if you are planning to give birth at home. They will help you interpret your body's signals.

One general rule is that you should call then go to the hospital when you have *regular contractions* that are *about sixty seconds* long and keep coming *every two or three minutes*. For those who have given birth before, it might be good to leave a little earlier, since the body's signals can be more varied.

You should also call the hospital if:

- Your waters break.
- You are bleeding vaginally.
- Your baby is moving less often or the pattern of movements has changed.
- You have a headache, visual disturbances or upper abdominal pain.
- You feel unwell, have a constant abdominal pain or have any concerns.

The Pushing Stage

This phase starts when the baby has finished the journey down the birth canal and has its head right at the pelvic floor. This can lead to an overwhelming, involuntary urge to push that takes over the body. Many women feel as though they are going to have a bowel movement or like there is a heavy pressure against their back-passage. However, some women have more diffused sensations that are harder to define. Some women feel overwhelmed by the contractions at this stage and therefore all they can do is to let their body take over and push. For others, it can be a less pronounced force, especially for those who have received an epidural.

The work of the uterus

The uterus, the pelvic floor and the abdominal muscles all participate in the pushing phase. The contractions press the baby's head towards the opening of the vagina, which increasingly gets wider with each contraction. The opening of the vagina works like an elastic band that widens around the baby's head. It is common for the baby's head to retract back after each contraction for a while; this allows the tissue to become more elastic. Finally, the baby's head has expanded the vagina to a point where the head does not retract after a contraction. At this point, it is common to feel a burning sensation on the perineum. This is a sign that the actual birth is very close. Once the head has stretched the opening to a point where it is wide enough, the baby's head is born, followed by the shoulders and the rest of your baby with the next contraction. This stage generally lasts anything from minutes to a couple of hours, often depending on whether you are a first time mum or have birthed before.

Emotions During The Pushing Stage

The pushing phase can be experienced as more tangible than the opening phase. The pain has shifted, and the contractions work more clearly to move the baby down and towards birth. This part of labour can give a sense of relief since you can actually feel that something is happening, though it can also feel frightening since the pressure may be intense. The pushing phase requires you to take an active part in the process and the challenge is to go along with it. The pressure on the pelvic floor can give way to the sensation that you need to go to the toilet to open your bowels. This might lead to you squeezing your muscles and working against your body. Just because you feel like you need to defecate does not necessarily mean that you will, and if you do, the staff will take care of it in a discreet way. Try to embrace the sensation and not hold back.

This is also the stage when many women think of the impossibility of something that big coming out of something that narrow. Just because you feel a certain way, however, does not mean that it is true. The vagina is made up of pleated mucus membrane. It is perfectly constructed to widen and let your baby through. You can picture how it hugs the baby and adjusts itself to the baby passing through. The opening of the vagina can stretch and become large enough to birth your baby, and after it will fold back again to its normal state.

You might be filled with energy since it is now obvious that soon you will finally meet your baby. You might become scared since the pressure can appear overwhelming, or it may feel wonderful that something is finally happening. The impulse to bear down can feel confusing since your body takes over and you find yourself incapable of holding back. You might get the feeling that you will not be able to go through with it, even though your body is working at top capacity. You may not find this phase easy, but you can, with the help of the four tools, give your body the support it needs so that you do not waste any energy working against what is happening.

Length of the birth

Each birth consists of all these phases, but each labour varies greatly in length and intensity. Some women never feel the early labour phase and start off their labour in the active first stage. Other women have a prolonged early labour phase. There are cases when the cervix opens to ten centimetres very quickly, only to come to a halt while the body takes a break and recharges before the pushing contractions begin. The opening phase might be very long and drawn out, only to be followed by a short pushing phase.

Even though it might be very difficult for us to acknowledge that there are areas of our lives that cannot be controlled, we must accept that we have no control over the process of childbirth. As a rule, however, a first-time mother has a longer labour than a second-time mother. The second baby usually comes quicker. There are exceptions, as always, and you should keep an open mind to whatever unfolds. The goal is to manage the labour by handling *one* contraction at a time and by taking advantage of the rests in between, regardless of which phase you are in. Nevertheless, the length of the whole process can be of concern, both if it is very drawn out, or alternatively so quick that there is no time to get to the hospital.

Many women wonder how they will manage to get through a prolonged birth process, with hours upon hours of pain. A process like that will obviously tire you, physically as well as mentally. However, it is important to know that it *is* possible to rest, and even sleep during parts of the process, and this is especially necessary if your labour extends over several days. There is always a break between the contractions, as I mentioned before. There are many things that can prevent a woman from *accessing* and making the most of these breaks; these include fear, false expectations, feelings of excitement, stress reactions or simply a lack of understanding about how to rest and recharge.

Women are often *told* to relax, rest and sleep when labour starts, but it can feel impossible to do so. The art of knowing *how* to relax can be one of the most crucial preparations for the birth and can mean the difference between a positive and a negative experience. No techniques in the world will be of any help to you if your mental strength is spent. You will learn more about how you can sleep and rest during labour in the next section of this book.

The other side of this coin is if the birth happens too quickly; however, this is uncommon for first-time mothers. A very quick, short labour can be difficult to handle physically and emotionally, since from the start, contractions are intense and frequent, with short gaps between them. You might feel that things move too quickly for you to keep up and understand what is going on, which can be very stressful. If you do not become scared, however, you will find the strength to turn your focus inwards and get in touch with what is happening, regardless of how intense the experience gets. Most of the time, the body works perfectly and there is seldom anything wrong. If you feel you will not make it to the hospital or birthing centre on time, you might do best to stay where you are, in the car or at home, to get as good a birth experience as possible. Your partner or support person can stay in touch with the midwife or hospital via the telephone.

If you are very worried, talk to your midwife and make a plan for how you are going to deal with a quick labour and birth. It is better to be prepared than to worry about something you cannot control. In both of the above scenarios it is important not to fixate on how you imagine things will play out. Instead, stay focused on what is actually happening and make sure you know how to handle the contractions.

Exercise: Preparations for dealing with the length of the labour

Exercise

- In order to conserve energy, it is important to minimise stress and the production of adrenaline; this enables you to maximise the benefits of gaps between contractions to rest and recharge.
- Do not decide beforehand how long you think the birth is going to take, keep an open mind.

The Baby's Journey Out

1. During the latent and active first stage of labour, your baby prepares for delivery by resting its chin against its chest and turning its head into the correct position in the pelvis.

2. Your baby is ready to begin its journey outwards when the cervix is fully opened.

3. At this point, your baby is pushed down through the birth canal with each contraction. On its way through the vagina, your baby will turn in order to adjust to the shape of the pelvis and the vagina; it rotates and works together with you.

4. When your baby's head has reached the opening of the vagina, the journey is almost complete. When the head has made the opening wide enough, it passes through and your baby's head is born.

5. Sometimes the shoulders and body follow after the head with the same contraction. Usually, however, there will be a brief pause of a minute or two, then the shoulders and body will be born with the next contraction.

After the birth

After the baby is born, there is a break in the contractions before it is time for the placenta to be delivered. The break can last anything from a few minutes to about an hour. When the placenta has detached from the uterine wall, the uterus will contract in order to push the placenta out. The placenta is soft and flexible and it passes through the opening of the vagina easily. Usually the placenta and membranes are delivered by the midwife or doctor, who gently pulls on the umbilical cord.

When this stage is complete the midwife or doctor feels the abdomen to check the womb has contracted down, which is necessary in order to control further bleeding. Finally, it is important to gently inspect the labia, perineum and vaginal wall to see if there are any tears or lacerations that require stitches.

A mother is born

When the birth is over, your new life as a mother begins. It takes time to make this adjustment, both physically and mentally, and various emotions and feelings will come and go. You might feel elated, or you might find it takes a while to discover your mothering and nurturing instincts.

You will probably feel very sensitive and emotional after giving birth. This is because you need to be emotionally available to bond with your new baby. This emotional openness makes you vulnerable or a little bit blue. Therefore, you are not meant to meet too many people, or to be too active. If you wait a few days, you will have had a chance to bond with your baby and you will be a little stronger and more resilient.

The body can be sore after the delivery, and alongside this you may be starting to breastfeed your baby. This is also a bodily process that can take time to become confident with and to establish. Whilst breastfeeding can be a wonderful thing to do, it can also be difficult and challenging at times. You need plenty of peace and quiet.

Overcoming difficulties and solving problems will build your confidence as a parent. You are the mother of your baby and you have all the love and capacity you need to take care of him or her, even if you do not know all the details.

Do not hesitate to ask for advice or support when you need it and do not see this as any kind of failure. A positive outlook does not mean you never ask for help, but rather that you believe in your ability to handle what comes, even if things now and then are not working well.

Summary

Your body is designed for the physical experience of childbirth and the biggest challenge you need to overcome is to go along with it and allow your body to give birth.

- Fear is a normal and natural emotion, designed to protect you from danger.

- Your body reacts to fear by preparing to deal with a potentially hostile situation. You are supposed to evaluate the situation you are facing and if there is no threat, the alarm systems in your body will turn off and your body returns to its normal state.

- Problems occur when the danger appears to come from within your own body; in other words, when the pain itself is seen as the threat. What could be seen as threatening does not disappear; the stress reactions can then linger and will slowly break you down

- To avoid this, you must realise that it is the fear, not the pain that breaks you down. If you understand how your body reacts to positive, as well as negative, emotions you can enhance the positive and stop or reduce the negative ones.

- It is your perception of fear and pain that determines the stress reaction. This is called coping. The stress reaction will be reduced if you recognise fear and know how to face it and deal with it.

- Use the power of the feeling trust and positive energy to minimise the momentum of fearful emotions, to activate the inner physiological ability to give birth you have inside and your birth hormone oxytocin. If you have confidence in your ability to give birth and believe in the fact that there is a meaning to whatever you are going through, you can free up your body's ability to work as it is designed to and to lessen the pain. You will then emerge from the experience of giving birth as a stronger person, with a positive reflection on the journey

- Pain during childbirth serves a purpose and in order to further lessen the power of fear, you need to understand what that purpose is. Therefore, it is very helpful for you to understand the function and rhythm of the contractions. During the contractions you can utilise the four tools, described in the next part of this book, to help you cope with the contractions and maximise the rest periods in between.

- Accept that it is natural and normal for fear to periodically arise in labour and birth. However, learn to recognise it, face it and handle the fear by using the tools. This will ensure that fear does not escalate and take hold, with its resultant negative spiral of emotions and outcomes.

Gabriella's Birth Story

April 13ᵗʰ
00.00 am

I am at the hospital. Relax, I am here now. I like the room. The warm, friendly staff greet me. It only takes midwife Lina five minutes to 'get me'. What a relief! A midwife in training is right next to Lina. I say it is fine if she wants to stay. I am four centimetres dilated now. I change clothes. I stop and breathe into every contraction, sinking into it. It is not hard. We walk around, laughing and talking in between contractions. After half an hour, I want to retreat to the room and not see people. I just want to be cocooned in the comfort of the delivery room. Richard quietly takes on the role of the protector, coach and support person. We decided beforehand that I would use my hands to gesture when I feel a contraction. When I raise my hand, everything must go quiet and calm. Juice with a straw, water, pillows – he gets me whatever I need and keeps close to me. I cannot communicate with words – I need to sink deeply into myself. He understands. I feel how he is right there with me – not feeling excluded. It is priceless to know that I do not have to explain myself, or complicate things by saying 'Please, could you help me by...' because there is no way I could find the time between contractions. I feel the love and support from his hands when he massages my shoulders and firmly brings his hands down along my body. It calms me, brings me closer to the earth, gets the oxytocin flowing in me. I stay with the contractions. I manage them all on my own. I dare to sink into each contraction, dive in and momentarily lose myself. With each contraction, I say to myself 'Yes, baby, down, out, out, out and down. I love you and you are welcome into this world.' Suddenly, the pain intensifies – I can feel a barrier now. It is a barrier of fear, a deep fear from the bottom of my soul. It is mine and I must face it. I can see it; it has a shape to it. It is like a see-through floor, tinted red; I know I must go through it to see the ground, but I seem to bounce back without the ability to go through it. A moment of panic – I cannot go down. I dare not sink all the way! I know the only way to get this baby out is to dive even deeper into myself, to give in to the pain. I need the support of our doula, whom I know can help me through this barrier of fear.

02.00 am
My doula arrives at 02.00. She is all calm, strength and experience, and I trust her completely. The first thing she does after saying hello is to turn the radio off. 'Aha!' I think to myself, 'I was trying to escape through the music!' I must give this my all for it to work. The room is quiet now. My confidence returns and I feel safe as she touches me, caressing my hands and body. Softly and calmly, she guides me down into myself. She is there during each contraction and I can talk and think during the breaks in between now. I observe myself from a distance. The redness of the fear evaporates when she assists me during the contractions and I now see light as I close my eyes. The light is the right way to go. The pain is even more intense now, but I am completely calm inside. I manage to let go more and more. The atmosphere in the room is of great importance – it has to be absolutely quiet during the contractions for me to be able to go deep inside and disappear within myself. Something feels wrong though. The student midwife is giving off the wrong kind of energy. She is all revved up and her energy is not in sync with the grounded, calming mood I need to surround myself with. I feel bad, but I must express my feelings. I ask Lina the midwife if she can tell her student to stay back a bit. Lina understands completely and I let go of that thought. I am once again calm and peaceful.

03.00 am

Six centimetres dilated now. I discover that the more I am able to let my feelings, my body and my mind go, the easier it gets. I have the courage to find a position where I tilt my head back with my chin up towards the ceiling, as if I was utterly defeated. I let my arms hang loose, with my palms up, almost like I am meditating. This makes it easier for me to breathe through the contractions. I used to lean forward when the contraction came – like I was trying to protect myself or hide. Instead, I give in. Nothing else exists. Richard massages my back firmly during the contractions; it feels as if the baby is ready to come out through my spine.

I take a very hot bath. The sound of the running water helps me to let go of everything around me. Richard is positioned behind me with cold towels and ice water, ready to cool my forehead and chest between the contractions. My doula is right next to me, holding my hand through the pain, guiding me. The world is fading more and more.

I am completely calm and secure. I get all the help and undivided focus I need to be able to fold into myself. Every ounce of panic that surfaces is swiftly overcome by the strong and soft voice of my doula. During each contraction, she reminds me to relax with something like a mantra, 'Relax your eyebrows, soften your jaw, loosen your chin, relax your shoulders.' Richard starts chanting 'Yeeeeesss' in his deep voice. While all this is happening, it hits me how it almost feels like I am in a Tibetan monastery. The thought makes me smile. This deep, repeating chant helps me to stay grounded. I sing along with him, seeking the depth of his tone. The pain is shifting; it wants to move out and down. I need to stand up. I sit on the toilet for a few minutes. I welcome the contractions with my breath. It is 04.00 am. It is starting to bear down; I recognise the sensation. The pushing

*contractions are probably about to start soon. I move to the bed
and lean forward on a pillow by my belly. NOW, the excruciating
force overtakes me completely. I feel like I am about to explode. It
does not end. I cannot breathe. I just have time to think 'Help me. I
cannot take this any longer. I want gas and air.' My doula is repeating
'Yeeess, yeeeess.' Now all I can do is push, push, push out. I do not
use the Entonox; there is no time. Suddenly – that burning, piercing
pain. The head is fixed. I am holding on to Richard and my doula
for dear life. The pressure is immense. The force feels like it is ripping
me apart. Her words ring in my ears 'You can do this, everything is
alright, he is going to be here soon, push him out.' She repeats this
over and over again. Then 'SPLASH!' His whole body emerges in
one push. I hear a scream as warmth is rushing from me. The pain
is gone and I can breathe. I listen for him. I listen to everybody's
reactions. Is he whole and healthy? He has a short umbilical cord, so
they cut it. I get help to turn around. Our miracle is resting on my
chest. He is so beautiful! Were you the one inside of me waiting to
come and see me? My beloved son, welcome to this world!*

*I was only bearing down for 13 minutes, but it felt like an eternity.
At 04.18, 14 April 2008, out little prince was born.*

The four tools

In this part, I have picked out the four most powerful and effective tools whose purpose is to overcome fear and stimulate trust and confidence. Each of the tools you will learn in this chapter will help you to open up the inner capacity of your body and enable you to find your own way to give birth. The tools help you quickly and easily lessen the feelings that hinder the birth process and stimulate the ones that help it. They boost your self-confidence and your ability to deal with the contractions and the pain, so that the birth-giving experience becomes as positive as possible.

They will not necessarily take away all the pain or make the process of giving birth 'easy', but they will help you relax and make it easier for you to work with your body, and not against it, during labour. The tools enable you to stop fear taking over you; instead, you actively steer the body away from fear. When fear no longer receives all the focus, robbing you of all your energy, you have the ability to access the power within you; a power which will help you to give birth to your baby.

The opposite of fear is trust

In order to break the sometimes entirely automatic chain reaction that fear leads to, the tools in this book focus on the opposite of fear: trust. This is the *feeling* that the four tools stimulate. You feel safe and secure when you know that what is happening to you is not damaging or harmful. The body's 'peace and calm' system kicks in, the hormone oxytocin is activated, blood circulation increases to the reproductive organs, you gain more energy and you feel more secure and confident. Additionally, your breathing becomes softer and quieter, your muscles relax, your voice deepens and your thoughts calm down and become more positive. The feeling of trust also accommodates a natural balance between activity and recovery.

To be able to stimulate relaxation and trust, and thereby lessen the negative emotions which make the birthing process harder, the tools aim to use your body's own natural expressions of trust: gentle breathing, relaxed muscles, a deep voice and positive thoughts. All emotions have their own body language and way of manifesting themselves physically in the body. The tools make use of this natural neurological connection between your body language and your emotions. By allowing your body to express calmness and trust in each contraction, even when you do not feel entirely safe or secure, more emotions of trust, calm and wellbeing are triggered. These will, in turn, tell your body that *it is safe to give birth*, which in turn gives way to the *physiology of labour being activated.* You already have all these connections and abilities – all you have to do is show your body the way.

To illustrate this, I would like you to imagine having a contraction. When you start sensing the contraction, you might automatically tense up. This is a perfectly natural instinct, but by doing this, you risk ending up in a negative cycle. To change this, try to instead do the opposite, and relax *as soon as* you feel the contraction beginning. This might be the opposite of your first impulse, but if, despite the pain, you are able to breathe slowly and quietly, relax your jaw, lower your shoulders, use a deep voice and think positive thoughts, the feeling that you are under threat will not arise. You are guiding your feelings *away* from fear and *towards* trust and calmness. Instead of stimulating fear, you stimulate trust.

By doing this, you swap a negative spiral for a positive one. By allowing your body to express the opposite emotions from fear, you create as big a distance to fear as possible and make it more difficult to fall into the negative spiral. This is how easily the tools work. The paradox can be that at the same time as they seem so simple, they can be quite challenging to use. It requires both courage, training and knowledge to learn how to go against your initial instincts, and relax, in what can sometimes feel to be a difficult and frightening situation. However, when you finally take the steps needed and feel the difference, you will not look back.

Pain can trigger an automatic chain reaction that can manifest in the following ways:

1. Pain.

2. Reaction: Tension, saying 'No', wanting to escape.

3. Result: Body resisting and fighting against the birth and blocking the physiology.

You can break this chain reaction and stimulate positive feelings by rejecting your first impulse with the help of the four tools, and instead do the opposite:

1. Pain.

2. Reaction: Relaxing, saying 'Yes', staying in the moment, letting your body's physiology unfold and work as it is designed.

3. Result: Working with your body and gathering confidence to give birth

Physical expressions of fear vs. Trust

When I started working with labouring women, I discovered how many times they were unaware of the negative stress pattern they were caught up in. I learned that I could recognise it by studying their *body language*. As time went on, I developed an ability and sensitivity for interpreting their body language and this became instrumental in helping these women.

To be able to use the four tools, you need to understand how fear manifests itself in the body. Once you have *recognised* emotions that will hinder the process of labour and birth, you are then in a position to change them and break their hold, and halt the accompanying negative reaction cycle. However, it is not enough to only recognise the negative reactions. You also need to be aware of the positive reaction patterns, since the tools are based on them, and you need to deepen and protect these emotions. With this in mind, here is a short run-through of the most common body signals for both of these emotional states:

Fear and stress

Fear and stress can manifest in one or in a combination of several of the following ways:

During contractions

- Loud and forced breathing.
- Clenched jaw, tense shoulders and hands, general bodily tension.
- Fluctuating gaze and difficulty staying still.
- Tendency to push up with the hands and tightening the thighs while lifting the body upwards.
- Standing on tiptoes.
- High-pitched and strained voice.

Generally, and also in between contractions

- Difficulty relaxing.
- Difficulty sleeping and resting, sometimes for several days.
- Negative emotions and resignation that persists.

Trust and confidence

Trust, safety and confidence can manifest in one or in a combination of several of the following ways:

During contractions

- Calm and quiet breathing.
- Heavy and relaxed body.
- Closed eyes or focused gaze.
- Willingness to allow the contraction to flow through the body, and not to control or fight it.
- Deep and calm voice.

Generally, and also in between contractions

- Relaxed and centred between contractions.
- Ability to sleep and rest when tired.
- Positive and neutral emotions that come and go naturally.

The birth without fear tools

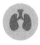 **BREATHING**
Your *breathing* is directly connected with your feelings. By breathing *calmly* and *quietly* you will create a positive feeling, which reduces stress and fear.

 RELAXATION
Relaxation is the opposite of escape and will help you to stay calm throughout your contractions. This will reduce tension and prevent you from working against the contractions, which would hinder the birth process.

 VOICE
Your *voice* can be of great help in preventing fear. A *deep* voice will lessen stress and fear and also engage your abdominal muscles, which will assist you during the pushing phase.

 THE MIND
The *power of the mind* can help you access your inner resources of optimism, trust and faith. These resources will be there for you during labour and for when you are facing pain.

How to use the tools

The tools can be used throughout the whole labour and birth journey whenever facing a contraction regardless what phase you are in. You can imagine them as steps on a staircase that you slowly walk down during labour. When the contractions come during the early stages of labour, you might start by only working with the breathing and relaxation. As the contractions become more intense, you take the breathing and relaxation with you down to the next step, which is your voice. The voice will assist you to stay calm, helping you to relax your muscles, and alongside this you may require the added assistance of the power of your mind. When you have walked down all of the steps, the tools will blend well together. You may also use only one of the tools during your whole labour; they all work very well on their own. I have heard of many women using for instance, the voice from early labour on. Regardless which tool you use, the four tools will lead you towards trust and your goal: welcoming your baby into this world.

You might get the impression that these tools are simple and obvious when you practise using them during your pregnancy. However, what might seem simple and obvious now can be difficult and easy to forget when we are scared and overcome by fear. With this in mind, do not underestimate the importance of practising using them.

Some tools may feel quite comfortable and natural to you and others might feel more alien. Do not be afraid of the ones that feel strange or unfamiliar at the moment. Sometimes, what works best during labour might be something you thought you would not use at all! Remember that your everyday body is not the same as your birthing body. In labour it can be hard to intellectualise the reasons why the tools work; you will simply feel that they do.

Meeting the contraction

The tools presented in this book will help you to activate the body's own pain inhibitors. This system is there to help you, and it kicks in when you feel trust and safe. However, if your focus is only to lessen or *stop* the pain you are feeling, these techniques could have the opposite effect and instead work against the whole birthing process. The body works better if you are accepting and welcoming of the contractions. It is normal and natural for the contractions to become more intense as labour progresses. This is necessary, as it is a sign of the uterus working as it is designed, working towards giving birth to your baby.

An essential insight is that each contraction always stands for something *positive* – the birth of your baby– even if it does not always feel like it does. If you are trying to slow down or halt this force, you end up working against your body. Instead of making you feel stronger, it will make you lose faith in your own ability. To avoid this, your preparation needs to include strategies to handle the contractions. Meeting or receiving the contractions means to allow them to come. The tools help you to go along with a set of events that you cannot control and they also allow you to prevent the conflict that may arise within your own body. They let you receive the pain and view it through a less negative lens, despite the force of it increasing through the stages of labour until your baby is born.

I was present at a birth where the woman was afraid to move around. The pain got stronger every time she shifted position. She took a bath and became more and more motionless. I encouraged her to move around, even though it was more painful for her and we made up a plan to help her to deal with the contractions. Rather than tensing up, she would go along with them and embrace the movement. When the contractions came, I encouraged her to welcome them. I kept repeating that everything was as it should be and that her body was helping her to reach her goal. She stepped out of the bath and as soon as she felt the contractions, she put her head back, made a deep sound with her voice and swayed her hips slightly. It worked! This made her feel powerful and self-confident, since she had discovered, with the help of this simple practise, the ability to face and handle the contractions and the pain.

Handling the contractions with the four tools

You cannot *control* the birth process, how it will feel, when it will start or finish, or whether it will be a long or a short one. You can guess of course, but at the end of the day you can never control or foresee it. However, you do know one thing; that the process will *start* with contractions, and it will *end* with contractions. You also know that each contraction is one step closer to you meeting your baby. So, to help your body and to create a feeling of positive control, you and your partner, or any other support person, can focus on handling *one contraction at a time,* by using the four tools. After each contraction comes a very important rest. These two events make up the rhythm of the birth process, and it is up to you and your support person to use both to your advantage. The rest is *just as* important as the contraction, as you and the baby cannot do one without the other.

Think of the contractions and the rest like the waves in the ocean. Softly and steadily you follow the flow and rhythm of birth by flowing with the contractions, down in the body with the least amount of resistance, allowing them to do their important job, and then you surf up again onto the top of the wave where you and your baby can rest.

It is important to agree with your birth partner on a sign for when the contraction begins *and* for when it ends. A simple word such as 'now', lifting your hand, or just a gentle squeeze of your hand on your support person works beautifully. During the contraction you then work together with the four tools to guide the body away from fear and back to safety. When the contraction ends, you can signal this with a sigh, which also functions as the beginning of the important break. I will discuss the sigh in more detail when I explain the first tool, breathing.

BREATHING

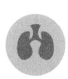

I had been hired as a doula for Mia and Adam. When I arrived at their apartment, I discovered that Mia had not slept for twenty-four hours. She told me that she was extremely tired and exhausted. She kept repeating this over and over, and I could sense her desperation. I watched Mia as she was having a contraction. She was sitting down on a chair, with another chair facing her. She took many deep breaths that could be heard throughout the whole room. I could see how her breathing pattern created fear in her body. The typical signs were there; her body was restless, her toes were curled in, her brow furrowed, her shoulders up high and there was a general sense of tension throughout her whole body. I moved very close to her, leant my forehead against hers and I whispered that she needed to adjust her breathing. During the next contraction, I talked to her softly, using a deep voice and I explained her that her breathing was too loud, and that she needed to breathe softly and calmly. I told her that I would assist her in breathing quietly. I stayed right there with her and as soon as I heard her breathing becoming forced, I reminded her to breathe softly and quietly. Slowly, her breathing adjusted. Her breathing became more and more silent, and she let each exhalation pour out from her body without a sound. The whole time, we worked together, with the aim of making Mia's breathing calmer and more passive and her body more relaxed. Before long, Mia was able to feel the results; the contractions grew gentler and she was less scared. She was fascinated and surprised at the difference. I continued to guide her and after a while, she felt such a big difference that she was able to fall asleep.

She rested for a few hours, and when she woke up established labour had finally kicked in. Her contractions were forceful and when we got to the hospital, she was six centimetres dilated.

Breathing is closely connected to your feelings and all emotions are manifested in your breath. You sigh when satisfied, gasp and hold your breath when scared, and start hyperventilating when you feel you must escape. The most noticeable signs of fear during labour often get expressed through a woman's breathing patterns. It is common to take a sharp breath in when a contraction comes, like you do when you get scared, or to take deep, noisy breaths. Many women believe intense, audible breathing is soothing and that it is important to oxygenate the blood for the baby as much as possible. However, the balance between oxygen and carbon dioxide is sensitive and gets disturbed by forceful breathing. Forceful breathing makes the pain and stress become more intense and this in turn creates anxiety. Anxiety leads to hyperventilation, which leads to more anxiety – a vicious cycle is created.

In order to change this behaviour and break this negative pattern, you need to find your way back to a natural way of breathing. Focusing on and slowing down your breathing is the most effective tool when it comes to lessening the fear and building trust.

Natural breathing

The most important elements of natural breathing are that it should be soft, quiet and without tension. Your breathing is calm and mild when you feel relaxed and safe. During inhalation, you use the muscles to fill the lungs. This is the active part of breathing. The exhalation is more passive; the air streams and flows out without you having to use any muscles and the exhalation is soft and quiet. As the air flows out of your lungs, your shoulders automatically drop and the rest of your body relaxes.

By breathing in a calm and relaxed way during labour, the body will find its organic breathing pattern, which will keep stress reactions and fear at bay. You do not need to put much effort into this, since organic breathing comes naturally and automatically.

Quiet breathing

While you are in labour, the *way* in which you breathe does not really matter all that much, as long as it is *soft* and *quiet*. If you are breathing in this way, your body will take over and create its own rhythm. It does not matter whether you inhale through your mouth or your nose. In my opinion, the more you think of how to breathe, the more difficult it becomes. Your body will find what works best for you, depending on how the baby is positioned and how deep or shallow you need to breathe.

A woman once told me she thought it was hard to breathe soundlessly during her contractions. Her *instinct* was to breathe forcefully and strongly. This raises an important point, which is that the four tools can be used to specifically influence and redirect your instinctive response. It is *fear* that is connected to the fight-or-flight response that kickstarts your breathing reflex. The purpose of rapid, forced breathing is to oxygenate the muscles of your arms and legs as much as possible; this is done in rapid preparation for a fight for survival, or taking flight and escaping danger. The uterus does not need the same amount of oxygen during contractions, as the work of many muscles working at the same time in your body. The increased breathing only serves to build more tension and fear.

You counteract this reaction by simply *choosing* to breathe softly and quietly. This will make it harder to tip over into stressed and forced breathing and ultimately lose control. The instructions to keep your breathing totally silent is not more difficult than the exercise below. This exercise will help you to learn to listen to your breathing so you can easily guide it to silence. Of course, you might wheeze slightly, but the feeling should remind you of a quiet wind, blowing in and out of your body. Let the breath flow freely. *The most important thing is to listen. If you can hear your breath, try to make your breathing as quiet and as soft as possible.*

If you find it difficult to breathe slowly, you might want to increase the speed of your breathing until it feels comfortable – but remember to keep it soft and quiet. Do it your own way if you have difficulty following the instructions, but always remember the basic principles of *'soft and quiet'*. Go back to your normal, natural breathing when the contraction eases off. If the intensity of the contraction makes it impossible to breathe softly and quietly, you can start using the third tool; your voice. Making a sound while exhaling helps you avoid falling into a forced breathing pattern during the more difficult moments of a contraction.

Exercise

Working consciously with the breathing cycle can make the breathing feel strained and uncomfortable. Do not get hung up on trying to change things; rather, try to simply *explore* and *observe*. Focus on relaxing and feeling comfortable.

STEP 1. If you listen to your breathing while reading this, you can get a sense of how it sounds when you are unafraid. Put the book down and observe *how* you are breathing. How does it sound? Are your inhalations and exhalations loud or quiet? *Where* in your body can you feel your breath? What happens when you inhale? What happens to your body and shoulders when you exhale? Repeat this a few times.

STEP 2. Try breathing *loudly* and with *force*, so that you can hear your inhalations and exhalations in the room. Exaggerate a few breaths. Notice how this changes your feelings. How does your body feel? How long can you keep going before you start to feel dizzy? What is the biggest difference in comparison to the quiet breathing?

STEP 3. Go back to the quiet, calm and soft breathing. Let your exhalations be slow, pleasant and soft. Breathe in a way that feels comfortable and good. Repeat this a few times. Notice how this makes you feel emotionally. How does your body feel?

Ask your support person to listen, so that he or she also can hear the difference between the two types of breathing.

Techniques during contractions

These techniques can be used for the entire length of the contraction:

1. Inhale softly and quietly. The purpose of this is to simply keep your shoulders and upper body from lifting up, which they would automatically do if you take in too much air.

2. Exhale slowly and quietly. Exhalations are naturally longer then inhalations. It is during exhalations that your body sinks downwards and relaxes.

Finish the contraction with a sigh

We sigh with satisfaction and relief because it feels good. When you are relaxed and secure, you sigh several times per hour without hardly noticing. When you sigh, your shoulders drop and the muscles in your neck and face relax. This important function does not occur when you are stressed or scared. In today's hectic society, bodily aches and pains are common. This is because stress blocks the body's natural system for relaxation, recovery and rest.

You can use the sigh as a natural way of relaxing during labour. After the contraction has finished, it can be hard to get rid of any built-up tension. If you keep unconsciously tensing up after the contraction, it can be difficult to rest properly. By *sighing* after *each* contraction, you can neutralise the tension and relax the body. By doing this, you also create a downward movement which automatically makes the body more relaxed; you are using the body's inbuilt, natural system for relaxing.

Exercise

Put down the book and feel what happens when you sigh. Try slowly filling your lungs and then sigh with, and then without making a sound. You can try making a sound with an open or closed mouth, like a 'Haaa' sound, or some other sound.
What happens to your shoulders, your face and your arms when you sigh? Can you make the movement more pronounced? Try this a few times.

Technique after the contraction

Finish each contraction by filling the lungs and then exhaling with a deep sigh one or two times. The sigh can be soundless, or you can make a 'Haaa' sound. Do not be afraid to exaggerate the sound! Allow your shoulders to relax *down* and becoming *heavy* when you exhale.

RELAXATION

I was working on the maternity ward as an assistant nurse and went to visit Lena and Matthew. Lena had been labouring for over twenty-four hours, and she had not slept at all during that time. She was inhaling gas and air when I entered the room. During the contractions, she was getting up on tiptoes and her whole body was pulling upwards. Lena kept repeating how tired she was and how she wanted to rest. After a while, I felt like we had a connection and I suggested that she did things a little differently with the next contraction, so that she could get some rest. I encouraged Lena to let go of the gas and air for a short while, but that she could come right back to it if she didn't like what we were doing. She found it a little frightening to leave the Entonox at first, but tiredness made her ready to try almost anything. I closed the blinds and turned off the lights. I helped her to get on to the bed, with a pillow behind her neck, and then we began. As the contraction came, I helped Lena to slowly slow down her breath and become heavy, and to sink down into the bedding. With every breath, I talked to her about daring to get heavy and relax her shoulders and jaw. I kept encouraging her to remain heavy and relaxed as the contraction started. I made sure her breathing was soft and quiet and that it stayed that way throughout each contraction. All the time, I repeated 'heavy... heavy... heavy. Let your body go and feel yourself getting heavy... heavy... heavy.'

It only took a few minutes until we felt the calm, silent magic in the room. She lay there, completely still and beautiful. I knew her body still felt the pain, but also that the pain had changed 'shape'. Lena was now capable of being still, letting the

*forces inside her work. No movement or struggle could be seen
on the surface. As the contractions were no longer noticeable
her partner feared that they had subsided. I whispered that
they were as strong as ever, but that she was now able to accept
them. He was amazed and impressed by her ability to handle
them. After trying the new way of breathing and relaxing for
three contractions we agreed to continue with this method. Lena
gave me a wonderful explanation of how she was experiencing
the difference; she said in a deep, calm voice, 'It is fantastic! It
feels like the contractions are blowing through me now. Before,
it was as if they were tearing at my insides, but now they are
more like a soft breeze. The pain is still there, but it is softer.' Soon
she was able to rest, and was even falling asleep in between the
contractions.*

The foundation of all relaxation is the feeling of being heavy.
It is important learning to counteract stress and tension by
experiencing the downward *weight* of the body. The feeling of
heaviness will help you to stop fighting the contractions; instead
you allow your body to follow, and sink in to each 'wave' they
create. It is the weight of the body that will help you stay in the
moment and prevent you from trying to 'flee' and escape the
contractions. It is after all much harder to 'flee' when you weigh
a ton, than if you are on tiptoes, ready to run and take flight. By
feeling the weight, you will get a sensation of melting into and
becoming one with the contraction and it will stop your thoughts
from buzzing and distracting you.

One of the goals of the tools is to help your body take full
advantage of the contractions. When you are scared, you stay
on the defensive and block the body. Fear makes you stand on

your tiptoes, pull your shoulders up and tense your jaw. This focuses energy *upwards*, which is in the opposite direction to the contractions and birth process; hence, this makes it more difficult to give birth. The common denominator of the tools is that they work in the same direction as the contractions, which is downwards. Birth conforms to the law of gravity and moves in a downward direction. The baby moves downwards and the uterus actively works to help the baby on its journey downwards in your body. The contraction has a direction because its purpose is to push the baby out of the uterus. This tool will help you to reinforce this downward movement, rather than working against it. The goal is to have the least amount of resistance in your muscles so that you work together with the contractions, so that you instead use all your energy to support your body and baby.

Being actively passive

You need to allow yourself to be *passive* and *heavy* during the contractions; this will help your body go along with the downward movement of the birth. It is in this heaviness that the birth can take place. In order to find the courage to become heavy and passive, you need to work actively. It might sound contradictory to be passive and active at the same time, but using the tools is actually an *active way* of ensuring that your body is *passive*. In other words, it is by doing *nothing* and being passive that you allow your body to work in the direction of birth. By creating a mental image of sliding softly to the bottom of the contraction, it can make it easier to follow.

Diving technique

The Swedish midwife Cayenne Ekjordh has created a technique called the 'diving technique'. She had been working as a midwife for many years when one day whilst on holiday, she found herself overcome by a strong current and big wave in the Atlantic Ocean. She struggled desperately, but soon realised that this was all in vain. Caught in the middle of a wave she realised she had to let go and allow the wave to carry her towards the shore. It worked! She was bewildered and breathless, but she had survived. A few years later, she reflected on this experience and realised that this could be the way to handle the 'waves' of the contractions; if the labouring woman lets go and gets heavy, the 'wave' will eventually carry her to the shore. Cayenne's experience led to her creating the 'diving technique'. This technique encourages the woman to 'dive' into her body and the birth process without fighting it. It is based on surrendering and being passive, which allows the power of the wave-like contraction to do its work. I was inspired by the diving technique when I created the first two tools in this book.

Muscle tension

As previously mentioned, the body reacts to fear with a chain of automatic responses; you raise your shoulders, you clench your fists and tighten your jaw. Tension also shows in the face, as a furrow between the eyebrows and as a tightening in the lips and around the mouth. You are often not aware of these bodily changes and they can linger long after the contraction has ended. This is also how we are used to seeing birthing women on television and in movies! However, this is a picture of a woman in fear, not of a woman giving birth.

The trapezius muscle – the muscle that extends over the neck, shoulders and part of the back – is very sensitive and reactive to fear, our emotions and to stress. When you are exposed to something you perceive as threatening, your emotions are activated, the fight-or-flight response and defence is triggered, and the trapezius muscle is automatically affected.

You can break this automatic chain response by *actively and consciously* working to *relax* the furrow between the eyebrows, your face, shoulders, hands and the entire body during the contractions. By consciously relaxing in these muscles, or being heavy, you eliminate the flight response. To give a clear picture of what I mean by being heavy and passive, you can imagine the sensation of sinking into water. You get heavier and heavier with each breath. Practise experiencing a feeling of passiveness and weight in your body in different physical positions, such as standing up, sitting and lying down.

During each contraction you should sink deep down. Lean your head against someone or something, let your arms and shoulders sink, and relax and soften your face. When standing keep your feet hip distance apart so that you have a stable base, and rhythmically bend your knees so that the movement is down towards the ground. Use your exhalations to relax more and more. Be especially mindful of your shoulders, as they are prone to lift and become tense.

Exercise

Lie down or lean back on a chair. Tighten and then relax different muscles to get a sense of the difference between a *tense* and a *relaxed* muscle.

STEP 1

Tense and then relax two or three times:

1. Forehead/eyes
2. Jaw/mouth
3. Neck/shoulders
4. Arms/hands
5. Thighs/bottom
6. Feet

STEP 2

1. Tense your entire body. How does it feel? What emotions surface?
2. Use your exhalations to reinforce the downward movement. Start off by tensing your whole body. As you breathe out, let go of your jaw, head and shoulders. Let your arms and hands fall and let your whole body relax.
3. Repeat a couple of times and feel how all the stress melts away. How does it feel? What emotion does it produce?

Technique during contractions

When the contraction comes, you stay still or lie down.
Lean against something or someone, like your partner or
support person. Surrender completely downwards.

1. Relax your face, your brow and let your jaw
    hang loose.

2. Relax your shoulders and let them fall down, lower
    and lower.

3. Relax the rest of your body and let your arms,
    hands, bottom and legs sink down; let gravity
    take over.

4. Repeat the words 'heavy, heavy, heavy' in
    your mind.

5. Use your exhalations to relax even more.

Relax especially in your:
Brow/eyes
Jaw/mouth
Neck/shoulders
Thighs/bottom

Muscles of the pelvic floor

There are many muscles that make up the pelvic floor that might be tense during labour, without the labouring woman being conscious of it. If they become too tense, they can make the birth more difficult. Many of the muscles in your body are interconnected. This means, for example, that the muscles in the pelvic floor tense when the ones in your face, jaw and mouth are tense as well. You can utilise this connection to help the pelvic floor to relax by relaxing your face and jaw during the contractions.

Pelvic Floor Exercises

You can feel the connection between your muscles if you tense your pelvic floor muscles as much as you can and try to speak at the same time.

1. Squeeze and lift the muscles of the pelvic floor.
2. When you tense as hard as you can, try to speak and see how your mouth, jaw and cheeks feel.

THE VOICE

I was at Lottie and Philip's house working as a doula. The contractions had started with great force. Lottie was a little tense and I suggested she take a bath. The warm water surrounded her body as she sank down into the tub. There, she became aware of her breath and the weight of her body, and she was able to relax. We continued in this way, with the contractions coming and going. With time, they became more and more intense and she was having trouble giving in to them, even though she was breathing quietly and focusing on being heavy. She started shifting restlessly in the bath. She could no longer remain calm during her contractions. I could see the panic in Lottie's eyes and the fear of not having the energy to continue. She worked hard at relaxing, but I could see it was not helping her. When I looked at her I saw an image of something imploding, a strong internal force. During the contractions I noticed her making a noise and I heard clearly how her body was trying to create a sound. Yes, the sound! The sound would help her face the pain! Lottie's body knew this, however her fear was stopping her from realising it. I leant in and whispered that her body needed something extra to help and that I would help her explore what that something was. I slowly guided her to let her exhalations grow into a sound. I explained, 'When the contraction comes, I want you to let the contraction become a sound. Open your mouth and make a deep sound all the way from your stomach. Follow the sound and the force down your body and make a deep sound. Good, that is great, keep going.'

Slowly, Lottie started to greet the pain with sounds. Her voice grew deeper and deeper and she opened her jaw wide, letting the sound come from deep within. The whole bathroom vibrated from her deep sounds. Her voice made the contractions more manageable. Lottie had suddenly found what she was looking for, something to help her through the last intense work the body needed to do. She stopped fidgeting and she managed to sink down and remain relaxed. The difference was huge! Her contractions were strong and moving along, she kept making sounds and her partner helped her. The acoustics in the bathroom amplified the noises and it sounded like a concert! She also used the sound during the second stage of her labour and it helped her to push her beautiful baby out.

It can be very difficult to remain soundless during the last part of the opening phase, since the body is working hard during this very physical process. During the second stage of labour, the pressure on the pelvic floor intensifies as the baby moves further down the birth canal. One way of assisting the body in this work is to make sounds. The body often needs to release sounds. We can use sounds to express and let go of what we are feeling; for example, we laugh when we are happy, cry when we are sad, yell when we are angry, and we use deep sounds and sighs when satisfied. In sport, athletes often release a sound to help their body work at its optimum. For example, in shotput this happens as they release the shot, and in tennis as they hit the ball with the racquet.

For the body, creating a sound is a way of releasing some of the pressure, and many women feel they need to make sounds during labour. It is freeing, can feel good and it can also help you let your body take over. Making sounds can therefore be a helpful way to handle the pain during the later parts of labour. Some may feel embarrassed about making too much noise, but the physical impulse to do so during labour can be an extremely powerful tool; try to see it as a natural part of the birth process.

The deep pitch or tone of voice also has the benefit of engaging the necessary pelvic floor muscles that you use during the pushing phase. These muscles are an additional help to the baby to aid its descent, as it travels down the birth canal as a result of the abdominal pressure from above. The abdominal muscles consist of both horizontal and transverse muscle fibres, and within the pelvic floor there are muscles that can both contract and relax at the same time. The pelvic floor has been created like this in order to help the baby descend. By embracing a deep pitch as you sound, you are helping the body to slowly allow the baby to pass, as this activates the pelvic floor muscles to stretch and relax.

Using a deep pitch for the voice

It is less likely that you will freeze up and get scared if you use a deep tone of voice, since this pitch does not activate the emotional reaction associated with a high-pitched voice. If you do not feel safe during labour, your tone of voice will be high, causing a lot of energy to get lost. This high, tense voice relates to the fight-and-flight response, which tenses your muscles. When you scream in a high voice, you stimulate fear and block your body's ability to labour and birth. A *high pitch* sets off a *negative* chain reaction; the voice stimulates fear, which leads to muscle tension, which results in more fear and so on. By breaking this destructive cycle, you can facilitate the body to work as it is designed for the birth process. If you instead use a deep, low tone of voice, you actively prevent stimulating stress and fear and instead help your body.

The deep, low-pitch notes also engage the muscles in the pelvic floor, help you bear down and activate the assistance of intra-abdominal pressure when pushing.

Exercise

It can feel a bit uncomfortable and unnatural to make sounds and use your voice, which is why it is a good idea to do this exercise *before* labour, so you can get a sense of how it may work for you. Just keep in mind that what might feel uncomfortable and strange to do in your everyday life, can work perfectly during labour. You can start laughing while doing the exercise, this is perfectly fine, laughter is welcome, even in birth.

1. Lie or sit comfortably. Pay attention to your breathing as you have in previous exercises. Make an 'Mmmm' sound with closed lips when you exhale. The sound should be even and last for as long as you exhale. Repeat this a few times.
2. Relax your jaw and lips. Add more focus to each exhalation and use a deep 'Aaaahh' sound, with your mouth slightly open. Do not force the rhythm of your breathing; use your own natural pace. Relax your shoulders. Repeat this a few times, slowly and calmly.
3. Try making the sound deeper and stronger. Can you feel your abdominal muscles when you make a deep sound?

4. Now explore how it makes you feel when using a high pitched 'scream' and saying 'Eeeeey!'. Repeat this a few times. What muscles are used? Does your throat get tired? Where does the energy go?
5. Go back to the low, deep voice. Repeat a few times. What sensations can you feel? Can you feel the energy and direct it downwards through your body?
6. Then try to lean your head back slightly, with a slightly open mouth and soft lips. Let the sound simply come out of you and keep your palms open. How does this feel? Repeat a few times.

Technique during contractions

1. When you feel a contraction coming, use a deep, low-pitched voice coming from your stomach. Remember not to force it, and to relax your jaw, lips and throat. The more sound you make, the deeper you make your voice. Make the sound uniform and soft and extend it for about as long as you exhale. But do not force the exhale to be too long.

2. The angle of your chin can make a difference. If you keep your chin close to your chest, the throat area can be restricted. You should therefore lean your head back slightly and 'open up'. Remember, however, to always try and see what works and feels best for you.

Sound and breathing

You can use the sound as a tool to help you with the intensity of the contractions at the end of labour, as well as a technique that assists you with the pushing stage. The sound can help to maintain a soft and steady rhythm of breathing, since it is often difficult to extend your exhalations in the final phase of labour. Remember to keep the sound soft, a deep pitch and not too loud. When the sound is used as a pushing technique, you can use it to flow down with the pressure, whilst at the same time activating the abdominal muscles that assist when bearing down.

THE MIND

As I started my shift as an assistant nurse, I walked into the room of a second-time mother who was about to start pushing. I had read in her birth plan that she was afraid that this birth was going to be a repeat of her previous labour, when everything had moved along fine until she entered the pushing phase, during which everything seemed to stop progressing. This resulted in an assisted birth being required and she did not want that to happen again. I observed her for a while; I could see how her body was readjusting as it prepared for the pushing phase. As I stood there watching her, I could see clearly how her body was shutting down. It was tensing and starting to pull upwards, instead of downwards. Her face, neck, thighs and jaw were rigid and tense. I tried to help her with my tools, but to no avail. I realised that she was facing what she feared the most. Time passed and her body was not able to access its power even though it tried. She was fighting hard to gain control, but her body was locked and unable to work. She was almost out of time by now. The staff were preparing for an assisted instrumental birth. I desperately wanted to help her, but I didn't know how. I had another tool that I had not presented to her yet – to say the word 'Yes.' But where am I going to find the courage to tell someone I have met only an hour before that it can work to simply say 'Yes'? She was probably going to ask me to buzz off! To simply say 'Yes' at a time like this seemed a little crazy, but I decided to take the chance.

While the staff were preparing for the assisted birth, I leant in towards her. 'You are going to think I am a fool, but I have a suggestion to help you dare to push. Would you try it for three contractions?' She nodded and I explained to her that I would like her to say the word 'Yes' when the next contraction came. She looked at me like I was a crazy person, but she agreed to try – she was willing to try anything at this point. Soon, her body signalled that it was time for the next one and when the contraction rolled in, she let out a weak 'Yesss.' I praised her, but I realised she needed more help to dare to use this tool to its full potential. I encouraged her to try again, but this time with her mouth open. When the next contraction came soon thereafter, I said 'Yes' along with her. She opened her mouth slowly and a strong and resolute 'Yeeeeeeeeeeeeeeeees' came out, all the way from deep within her. Her body pushed and a few minutes later her baby arrived. Both the midwife and the obstetrician were confused, and the woman seemed to not quite understand it either. I stood there completely amazed. The woman was overjoyed! She looked up at me. 'That was so strange. It felt like a string that just snapped! The muscles relaxed and just let the baby go. Thank you!' I stood there amazed and grateful and I realised I had found an incredibly powerful tool.

I will never forget the first day I used this tool. It was crucial for my understanding of the power of the human mind. Since that day, I have helped hundreds of women use this tool during many births and it has proven to be one of the most powerful tools you can use.

It is not just the word 'yes' that can affect one's mind though. Your mind can be used in many different ways. This has been a well-known fact for a very long time within cognitive therapy. You can use the power of the mind as a powerful unlocking mechanism. You can 'unlock' any mental block with the help of a positively charged sentence. During the pushing phase, for instance, you can use the word 'down' when you struggle to follow with the sensations of the pressure. This sends signals to your muscles to focus downwards, and it makes it harder for you to tense up. In order to mentally accept the pain of the contractions, you can use the word 'open' as a reminder to focus your energy on what is important. If you find yourself saying 'no!' during labour, you should consider doing the opposite and say 'yes'. It is said that your mind can be your greatest friend, or your worst enemy. Remember that you can move mountains with the power of the mind.

Say 'yes'

When overwhelmed by pain, it is easy to say 'no!'. This is automatic when you are taken by surprise and do not have time to adjust to what is happening. Sometimes, you may not be aware of your inner voice saying 'no', therefore making it difficult to counteract. Hence, it is more important than ever to say 'yes' when your feelings are negative. It may sound stupid and a bit crazy, but the word 'yes' directly engages parts of the brain to find positive emotions, faith and power. This is an effect associated with expectations. By saying the word 'yes' it prevents your body from going into 'resistance' and instead 'unlocks' physiology.

This tool activating the power of the mind helps you to say 'yes' to the birth, 'yes' to your body and 'yes' to your baby. It powerfully influences your inner strength and motivation to withstand the pain. The word 'yes' helps you to be accepting of the contractions and the phases of labour, as well as to generate trust and self-belief in what happens. This is very important when facing the force and power of childbirth.

During labour you can choose to only use the physical tools we have talked about. They work perfectly for coping with contractions and you will find them extremely valuable. However, it can also be very useful to try this powerful emotional and cognitive tool. By using it, you also combine different tools, since it can help you breathe calmly, relax your body and use a deep voice.

The power of the mind is powerful and wonderful when activated. However, it can be a difficult tool to implement when faced with pain, challenges and the unknown. Despite this, when women choose to begin saying 'yes' they often find that it works and they keep repeating this – inwardly and/or verbally – all the way up until the baby comes.

Many women wonder when to start using this tool. A rule of thumb would be to use it when you start to feel the urge to say 'no!', or when the negative thoughts begin to emerge. Saying 'no', 'I can't take it/do it/carry on!' *blocks* your inner ability to give birth and it also stimulates fear and stress. I often say that if you insist on saying no to the baby, try to instead say yes to the baby.

Exercise

To really understand the close relationship between words and the body, try the following exercises.
Nod/shake your head

1. Nod as you say 'no'. Repeat a few times.
2. Shake your head as you say 'yes'. Repeat a few times.
The difference between saying 'yes' and 'no'.
1. Put the book down and relax your jaw, shoulders, arms, bottom and legs.
2. Then start *thinking* 'yes' and then 'no' as if saying the words aloud in your head. Repeat a few times. Did you notice a difference?
3. Let your exhalations turn into a deep sound. Repeat a few times. With an open, relaxed mouth let the deep sound turn into a 'yes' in a low-pitched, deep tone. Let the sound last for as long as your exhalation. Repeat a few times. How did that feel?
4. Now say 'noooooo' and repeat this a few times. How did that feel? What was the difference?
5. Go back to slowly saying 'yeeeees' with an open, relaxed mouth, using your deep voice. Let your head tilt back just a little bit as you do so.

Technique during contractions

1. Softly and with a deep voice, say 'yeeeeesss' repeatedly in a rhythm that feels comfortable.

2. Tilt your head back slightly if that feels good. This posture helps you to stay open. However, remember to do what feels best for you

Affirmations

Your thoughts make up the foundation of your life. You create them both consciously and unconsciously, and they can either hinder, or they can be used to help. The thoughts come from within you and therefore you have all the *power to change* the negative ones that arise. When you consciously redirect your thoughts to take a more positive course, you are using *affirmations*. Negative thoughts can simply be *exchanged* for positive ones. If you keep repeating an uplifting, positive thought, your subconscious will recognise it as being genuine. In this way, you can mobilise your inner strength and your inner ability to generate wellbeing. Your body will accept this new state without questioning if it is real or imaginary.

You can use different affirmations other than the word 'yes'. For example, you could use 'down' or 'heavy'. An affirmation helps to keep worry at bay and reduces the activity level in the brain by keeping it occupied. When your mind is unable to create worry, it activates the 'peace and calm' hormone, oxytocin. For affirmations to work, they need to be *positive* and stated in the *present tense*. Never use the word 'not…' in your affirmations.

Do not be afraid to try this during labour, even if you do not expect it to work. The technique that is most effective during labour is sometimes the one you might least have expected to work for you. Use what you learned from reading about the previous tool (the voice); then simply use your voice to create a word.

Suggestions on words to use

- 'Yes'
- 'Down'
- 'Heavy'
- 'My baby'
- 'Open'

Exercise

Begin using affirmations that strengthen you. Deliberately choose positive thoughts rather than negative ones. This is what affirmations are all about. Use your affirmations throughout your entire pregnancy. Write them down in a notebook and keep it next to your bed. Repeat the affirmations a few times in the morning and again at night. Reinforce the positive expectation by actively building faith and trust.

Examples:

- I am strong and calm.
- I trust my body.
- I can handle the pain.
- I understand I am afraid, but I can handle it.
- I accept all my feelings.

Visualising

For a moment, I would like you to *imagine* your breath as a waterfall; this image will help you to bring your focus to the same downwards direction. You are *visualising*. The effect you get when visualising is similar to the effect you get when using affirmations. You can begin to link how the pain of the contractions opens the door for the baby, alongside the direction that your body is working – to bring your baby down and out. By visualising these images, you also activate emotions connected to them, which helps alleviate and manage fear and stress.

I attended a birth where the woman was finding the pushing phase difficult. The labouring woman had become unaware of how much she was tensing up. The midwife noticed that the woman's pelvic floor was white and tight due to the lack of blood flow. We started working with her breathing to help her relax and to increase circulation. I instructed her to imagine how the inhalation came from a place above her head, and how the exhalation ran through her like a waterfall, through her chest and belly and out through her pelvic floor. Breath by breath we worked with this visualisation and eventually she found a rhythm and a way to picture this waterfall inside of her. Ten minutes after we started, her pelvic floor became softer and more supple. By using her mind to visualise a helpful image, the tension within her pelvis had eased, allowing the birth to progress.

Technique during contractions

1. Visualise your inhalation coming from a place in front of and slightly above you.

2. Imagine your exhalation as a waterfall, softly and quietly running through your chest, belly and pelvis. Repeat several times at your own pace.

Using the tools during labour

During early labour

You might not need to focus a lot on the tools during early labour. It may be enough to listen to your breathing and check to ensure that you are relaxed during each contraction. Your support person does not need to work very hard at this point in the process, since you are probably capable of relaxing and going with the flow as the contractions come and go. It is important, however, that the beginning of childbirth is good, and that you can relax when you need to.

Some women can have an intense and painful experience in this phase. When this happens they need the support person to be an active participant from the very beginning. Stay in touch with your feelings and use all your senses when deciding what support is needed at any given time. Also remember to conserve your mental energy by distracting yourself for as long as you can, until the point when you need to focus to get through the contractions.

During active labour

You are likely to be now using the tools more and more, hence this requires a great deal of concentration. During *each* contraction, use the four tools to sink down and welcome the contraction, thus allowing the body to do its job. The present is the only thing that matters at this stage. Try not to think about the next contraction, focusing instead, on the moment in hand. As the birth process moves further along the support person will need to more actively guide, encourage and support, to the point where they eventually stay with you through each and every contraction.

By the time you are coming up to ten centimetres and fully dilated you might find it more difficult to breathe softly and calmly. This is when you can use your *voice* as a guide to keep the rhythm and control. At this stage many women begin saying 'no!'; they feel that they do not want to do this any longer and fear begins to take over. They may start to worry that they will not be able to handle the situation, which creates a sense of hopelessness. This is when it is time to use the mental tool of saying 'yes'. This is a very effective way to turn the negative thoughts around and of opening the mind to the idea of actually being capable of giving birth.

During the pushing stage

You can keep using the four tools during the pushing phase. Alongside this, emphasise the feeling of *heaviness*. The most important thing is to focus on the direction, letting the body sink downwards. For example, if you are kneeling it is helpful to sink *down* towards your heels when you need to push. Bend your knees if you are standing upright. If your legs are tired, you can lie down on your side, but keep your mind focused on sinking down. If you are sitting or lying on the bed allow yourself to become heavy and to sink downwards. Think or say the word 'down'. It is as if you are coaching the baby inside to go 'down, down, down you go'.

If you vocalise, you have a powerful tool with which to greet the contraction. Keep the sound deep and steady; it should be very different from a scream. If you use this technique while pushing, you might need to close your lips. This creates an 'Mmmmmm' sound. Remember to keep directing all the power down through your body.

Women can often get stuck in a negative pattern during this phase and it may feel impossible to break free from a certain behaviour. If this is true for you, choose to use the power of the mind once again and say the word 'yes'. This helps to unlock the body's ability to birth, as well as changing the whole emotional experience for you.

Pushing technique

There is a tendency for things to get a bit frenetic during the pushing phase. It is easy to get swept up in all the cheerleading and pushing. It might sound unbelievable, but it really is possible for the pushing phase to be totally calm. Many women need time to let go enough and find the courage to let the baby out. The muscles making up the pelvic floor need to be relaxed for the baby to pass through. If the pelvic floor is tense while bearing down, two strong forces are working against each other. Passage of the baby is so much easier when the muscles of the uterus push down from above, whilst there is minimum resistance from the pelvic floor below.

If all is well with you and your baby you do not have to bear down with all your strength from the beginning of the pushing stage of labour. Instead, you should be completely passive, until the point when your body takes over and you can no longer resist pushing. You run the risk of unconsciously pushing *too* hard if you feel overtaken by the force of the contractions. Do not get swept up in fear or go along with the forced feeling you might get when you get the impulse to bear down. Remain in the moment and take in how it feels if you remain passive and relaxed. In this way, you create a connection with the body's impulse to bear down and allow the tissues time to soften and stretch.

You might also find that your pushing contractions are weak and that it is difficult to 'find' the right muscles. It is not uncommon for there to be a little pause in the second stage of labour, or for contractions to become weaker. Often the contractions re-establish on their own; if not there are various strategies that the midwife can help you with. Regardless of the reason, you can still find the energy and the right technique necessary to keep going. Be brave and try different techniques and find your own way.

Exercise: Finding the Right Muscles

What you need to do during the pushing phase is to increase your intra-abdominal pressure and at the same time allow your pelvic floor muscles to relax. Below are a few exercises for you to practise locating these muscles and to get a feeling for what it is like to bear down.

- Use a deep voice. Close your mouth and feel the sound inside your mouth, throat and chest. Repeat a few times and see how it feels.
- Imagine you have to push a tampon out of your vagina. Try a few times and reflect on the sensation.
- A fun exercise to do and one that works remarkably well, is to arm wrestle. When you are trying to get your partner's arm down, you are using the correct muscle group. Do this a few times and take some time to reflect. Try doing it again, now adding the deep voice. Did you notice how that works much better? Try to also close your mouth and direct the sound down towards your pelvis.

Using the tools with pain relief

When using nonmedical analgesia – such as warmth, bath/shower, acupuncture, support, massage and many other methods – you can keep using the tools as you usually would. Warmth is a very effective way of stimulating security, calm and relaxation; it helps you resist tensing up and fighting the contractions. Wheat bags, warm water bottles, showers and baths are therefore all great for pain reduction. You can keep a cool, wet facecloth on your forehead in the hot bath, since you might otherwise get dizzy from the heat. You also need to remember to hydrate, as you sweat out a lot of fluid in the bath water.

If you use Entonox, known as 'gas and air', you need to take long, deep and calm breaths. Relax your entire body when you exhale. In between contractions, you can return to the calm, soft and unforced breathing.

If you use an epidural, you can use the *relaxation* tool, in order to stay in the rhythm of the process, both physically and mentally, and also to help your body become heavy and relaxed. Use the voice tool to help deal with the feeling of pressure; the sensation of pressure can be strong both during the first stage of labour and during the pushing stage in the second stage of labour.

Remember the importance and benefits of support, closeness, touch and everything else that stimulates security, regardless of what pain medication you use, if any.

Using The Tools If Complications Arise

In the case of complications, interventions or operations, the staff take care of the medical side of things, whilst you and your support person should focus on handling the contractions, along with any emerging emotions together. Continue leading your body towards trust in each contraction. You should also stay close to each other and maintain eye contact. Remember to keep the tone of voice as *deep* as you can. If you give birth via caesarean section, continue to focus on your breathing, relaxing the muscles, the tone of voice and your mindset. If possible your support person can be next to you, keeping a steady hand with slight pressure resting on you whenever possible, on the shoulder for instance, and speak in a soothing voice. Make sure not to let stress and fear take over.

It is possible to have a positive, calm and strengthening experience despite an unexpected turn or complications.

Mobilising and resting during labour

To facilitate the birth process, you need to shift gears between activity and rest. The upright activities of hip rotation and changing positions during birth promotes increased blood circulation, stimulates the contractions, as well as helping the baby to move down through the birth canal.

It can be very helpful to softly and rhythmically move the hips around during the contractions. The movement releases tension and can give you a lovely feeling. I once heard a midwife give a good description of the benefits of this; 'Imagine you have a ring on your finger – to get this ring off, you need to bend and twist it while pulling it towards you. This is exactly the way the baby needs to be moved down through your pelvis.' It can also feel beneficial to proactively do something with the pain and, through the action, feel some sense of power. You are participating and the movement is your guide. Swing from side to side or move like a belly-dancer. Let your head be slightly tilted back; this opens the jaw and helps you relax the pelvic floor muscles. Try out different movements and positions. Use the four tools and the thought of being 'heavy' while exploring the movements.

Use gravity to facilitate the work the body needs to do. It does not mean you have to stand upright throughout the entire birth, but you should try to avoid lying flat on your back as much as possible. Few women choose to lie on their back during childbirth. Most women instinctively feel that this would make the process more difficult and hinder their access to their own inner power. Lying flat on the back instantly makes it anatomically like working uphill, the circulation to the uterus decreases and it reduces the available room within the pelvis for the baby to negotiate. Therefore, try to find upright, on your side or forward leaning positions, or try to sit up a bit if you have to be on your back.

It can be a good idea to bring along some music. The music you find most helpful might not be in the style you first anticipated though. I attended a birth where the labouring mother had brought some soothing melodies with dolphin sounds. When we turned it on, the woman got angry and yelled at me to turn it off! It turned out the music did not at all match the way she wanted to manage the pain and contractions. She asked us to turn on the radio instead. By pure chance, Michael Jackson's song 'Bad' came on. The mother-to-be instinctively started moving her hips in rhythm with the music; we all broke out in a big laugh. Laughing through her pain, she exclaimed how this music was better suited for what she needed.

Movements that can help during the active phases:

- During a contraction move your hips and the rest of your body (with or without music), while thinking 'heavy, heavy' or some other mantra.

- In the event you have had an epidural you are constrained to minimal changes in position on the bed. You can try alternating lying on your right and left sides, so long as you achieve an even distribution of the medication that alleviates the contraction pain.

Rest

Early one morning I was called to the hospital to attend the birth of Janet and Thomas's baby as a doula. Two wrecks greeted me as I entered the room. Neither of them had slept for two days and Janet was having a hard time with the contractions. Thomas was literally breaking down right in front of my eyes. He was terrified that he would not be able to be the solid support he wanted to be and he was clearly distressed. I quickly decided they needed to sleep. I closed the curtains and turned the lights off. Gently, I got them to lie down head to head, on a beanbag. Slowly, I guided them towards calm, soft and quiet breathing. I encouraged them to give in and let go of all control. 'You do not have to do anything right now. Give in. Surrender. Everything is alright.'

The first signs of sleep came soon afterwards. I kept speaking, using a deep, calm voice. I soon heard deep breathing – they were both asleep. They had finally been able to let go and the much longed for rest came. Janet woke up during each contraction, but she managed to go right back to sleep as soon as the contraction had subsided. After forty-five minutes, they woke up refreshed. They were fascinated and surprised! They had not realised that being able to fall asleep, or resting, would be so important.

We kept working actively throughout the day. Janet was using the tools during each contraction. The birth process was moving along slowly and she was not dilating very much. By the end of the afternoon she was exhausted and I managed to help her rest once again. She gave in completely and quickly fell into a deep sleep. Suddenly, whilst sleeping, she started dilating extremely quickly. Since she was not afraid, she kept sleeping in between the contractions. She sat up during each contraction, looked at Thomas and I and said, 'Epidural?' We thought this to be more of a question, 'Will I be able to handle this?' We put our hands on her and said, 'It is okay. Everything is okay. Let go... heavy... heavy... heavy.'

Her whole body relaxed and she fell back to sleep. The next contraction rolled in after about thirty seconds and she sat back up again 'Epidural?' We calmly responded and put our hands on her body. She sank down, tilted back and fell asleep once again. We kept this routine going for the next forty minutes, after which she started to sense the urge to bear down. We realised that Janet was almost fully dilated. She got down on a mattress on the floor and crouched on all fours. Recharged with new energy, she used a deep voice to be able to keep up with the pushing impulses. Aided by the soft instructions from her midwife and the support from her partner, she peacefully pushed her baby out.

As crazy as this might sound, it is possible to sleep during active labour. If the birth takes a long time, it is in fact the most important aspect of the process. Sleep is at the opposite end of the spectrum from fear and stress. You will only be able to relax enough to fall asleep if you are feeling safe and have faith in the fact that what you are going through is not harmful in any way. If you use the technique of letting the body become 'heavy' and completely relaxed between the contractions, the body will sense how you are letting go of control. This is a signal that it is permitted to rest and sleep. It is vital for both the body and the mind to have time to recover and recharge if you are going to have the stamina to last through a long labour. No technique or tool in the world can be a help to you if you do not get to rest and recover in between the contractions.

Some labours are quick and there is no need to sleep. More often, though, childbirth takes time, especially if it is your first baby. Sleep is important for the hormonal system and it has a restorative function, useful for the entire body. Most importantly though, sleep is essential for your mental wellbeing, which also helps you when bonding with your new-born baby. Mental strength is also key when it comes to preventing negative thoughts from taking over. If the mind does not get any rest, there is a risk that you will develop symptoms of stress, such as lethargy, anxiety and resignation. These feelings can cloud you from seeing the significance of what is happening and lead to a negative view of the birth experience. No human being can stay awake for more than twenty-four hours without developing feelings of anxiety. Insomnia is by no means a part of the physiology of childbirth.

Obviously, you are not meant to snore your way through the entire process, but you should be able to take *powernaps* in between the contractions. The sleep I am talking about is not uninterrupted, but rather a state that sets in between each contraction. As labour progresses and the contractions come with shorter and shorter intervals, it might be uncomfortable to wake up every time a contraction comes, but it is still an important *resting period* for your body.

Sleep during childbirth

You need to *stop talking* in between the contractions to be able to fall asleep. Try to not think too much. Choose to remain in a relaxed state during *and* in between contractions, as this will make it easier to fall asleep. You will need faith in your body and courage to do this, but keep in mind that it will not make the contractions any worse. Remind yourself that relaxation will make the contractions more effective and will make it easier for you to rest or power nap after each contraction subsides.

Sleep Technique

- Turn off the lights and make the room dark or dimly lit.

- Lay down or spoon with your support person.

- Find a position where your head, neck and shoulders are relaxed. You might want to lie on your side or be half sitting.

- Your support person can give you a hand or foot massage. The movement should be rhythmical, monotone, calm and steady. Keep massaging the same place over and over.

> • During the massage, your support person can repeat a word or a sentence using a slow, soft and deep voice. Try one or a few words like 'heavy', 'relax' or 'let go'. The continuous motion of the massage and the mantra will diminish the brain's ability to register pain, allowing a trancelike state to set in.

Remember that we are talking about short powernaps in between contractions. It can take about twenty minutes until you are relaxed enough to fall asleep, so keep massaging, stay silent and keep the room dimly lit. When you feel as though you have regained some strength, you can work actively again for a few hours. I have seen a pattern emerge, where most awake periods last for anything from four to six hours, and most rest periods are about forty to ninety minutes long. A rest period is followed by an active period, and so on. Women who have faith in their bodies and the birth process sometimes fall asleep for short periods while sitting, and even standing up for a little while.

Resting and recuperating are also important for your support person. I am not suggesting that he or she should sleep for several hours (unless that is okay with you, of course), but rather that he or she gets short periods of rest in order to be able to support you better.

When the baby is born
Straight after the birth your oxytocin levels are higher than during any other period in your life; this is to facilitate you quickly bonding with your new-born baby. Therefore, the moments

straight after the birth are important and delicate in terms of bonding for the entire family. There are many factors that can disturb the delicate physiology of this situation.

Continuous skin-to-skin contact with your baby is important. It is also imperative that you get some peace and quiet, as well as enough space to process everything that has happened emotionally. Everyone around you should whisper or talk in quiet, gentle voices. Keep the lights dim, and those with you should show respect and acknowledge you, so that you as a new family can begin to accept this new reality. Therefore, you should ask for some time as a new family unit after the baby is born. This is your special and unique moment and it can easily be disrupted by practical details.

Peace and quiet, continuous closeness and touch are also important for breastfeeding; this is, after all, also connected to the important hormone, oxytocin. If your body's production of oxytocin is at its peak, your body will also recover and heal more quickly. When you do start breastfeeding, your nipples can hurt until they get used to the sensation and action of your baby sucking at the breast. The four tools can assist you with handling the discomfort that can arise whilst establishing breast feeding. It is also important to seek support to ensure you are positioning and latching your baby well in order to avoid any damage to the nipples.

You should therefore continue to facilitate the flow of oxytocin after your baby is born; this hormone continues being important long after the birth and for the rest of your lives.

3

Support during birth

During the years I have worked as a doula I have come to understand how important the support person is for a woman in labour. Part 3 is therefore aimed at both the mother-to-be and the support person. You, as a support person, have a *key role* to play in preventing and reducing worry and fear during the birth process. Continuous support during labour has been proven to decrease the likelihood of a caesarean section, shorten the birth process and, most importantly, facilitate a more positive birth experience.

For you, as a mother-to-be, the support person is extremely important. He or she is the anchor in a 'stormy sea', that has waves of contractions, and they will give you faith and stamina when yours is faltering. The support person is also the one to make you aware of the physical reactions created by fear and stress. You can see, therefore, that it is very important for the support person to also prepare for the birth. *Preparing together* will give the support person the confidence to guide you through the birth process and it will make you feel secure enough to follow.

Giving support

*It was a calm evening in June and I was out on a doula mission.
Fredrik opened the door for me. Petra was in the bathroom, on the
toilet. I walked in and made sure to quickly establish a connection
with her. I looked into her misty eyes and I observed her for a
moment; I could see how she was having difficulty focusing with her
eyes. I saw how her body was uncomfortable and I could hear her
loud breathing. I whispered that I was there to support her. Using a
deep, slow voice, I started to explain what was happening in her body,
how her body was working downwards and how she just needed
to follow this by becoming 'heavy' during the contractions and to
breathe quietly. When the contractions came, one after the other, I
was there for her. I encouraged her to relax her jaw and her shoulders
and to choose to become 'heavy'. By helping her to focus her eyes, I
encouraged Petra to stay in the moment.*

*I soon noticed that she was getting heavier, rather than fighting
the contractions. Her body was now working with the contractions.
Everything was progressing well and Petra stood up, supporting
herself on Fredrik and I. Fredrik massaged and rubbed her back with
downward movements to help her let go even more.*

*In this position, the contractions seemed to intensify and became
more powerful. Petra bent her knees and followed the direction of
the baby. After each contraction, we encouraged Petra to take a deep
breath and to sigh softly; this made it easier for her to rest and relax
in between contractions. The contractions became progressively more*

intense and powerful and soon the tools were not quite enough for her. She started repeating how tired she was and how she thought that it would not work. Despite all this, she kept breathing softly and her body was still heavy; she was coping physically, but mentally she did not quite have the energy anymore. I encouraged Fredrik to move closer and whisper in her ear 'I am here for you... you can do it... I am here for you... follow with... let go... I am here.'

They were standing very close together and he was right there for her. I could see how quickly he picked up on what she needed. He knew exactly how to talk to her and he was protecting her. Using a deep voice, he guided her through the contractions. The midwife and I were there to support the two of them. Sometimes, they needed our help when something new arose, sometimes they wanted to be left alone.

After a while Petra's urge to push became stronger and stronger. Together, we encouraged her to tune in to, and move with, the direction of the pressure and to discover her deep tone of voice. Petra found a pitch that worked for her and we helped her to remain heavy and to let her bottom move towards the floor or her heels.

The baby moved further down the birth canal with each contraction. By being fully present in the moment, Petra managed to let her body work at its own pace. There were several cries of 'no!' and 'I can't do this!', but we knew that she needed to express these emotions and we kept supporting her, as well as encouraging her to rest before the next contraction. Then, it was time! Petra felt the head and I will always remember her eyes, filled with wonder and gratitude. With each contraction the baby's head moved closer and closer and you could now sense in the entire room that Petra was ready to birth her baby. Instead of cheering, we whispered, encouraging and helping Petra to be strong and to allow her baby to *come. The room was quiet and calm. Suddenly, Petra stood up and the head emerged. The midwife guided Petra and soon after a baby boy was born.*

Receiving support during labour is extremely important and I cannot overstate the significance of the support person. *Support and security* beautifully combat negative feelings and stress reactions that can arise during labour and birth. It is crucial for the woman in labour not to feel alone, and to be confident that she is seen, acknowledged and respected. It is sadly possible to be in a room full of people and yet to feel completely alone. Having people around a woman in labour does *not* automatically mean that she is supported. There are many occasions when the people around her simply do not know what to do.

Supporting a woman in labour is not always an easy task. During the birthing process she will temporarily leave the world you normally share. She will enter a sphere where she may never have been before, but where her body knows precisely what to do. She goes through an amazing transformation and she needs your support in order to have the courage to enter this part of herself, allowing her body access to its ability to give birth. She often requires lots of love and protection and you need to help her block any negative patterns you notice emerging. By knowing how a birth normally proceeds and which stress reactions to look out for, you can have the knowledge and confidence to step in and guide her.

Labour might very well be an unfamiliar situation for you as the support person as well, and it is therefore not unusual if you do not *automatically* have all the crucial knowledge needed. This chapter will help you to be a better support for the labouring woman. It will give some practical advice and you will learn more about how to use the most valuable tools a support person will need – *massage and touch*.

You can read and use this entire book to get a sense of the bigger picture, or you can use this part only. My wish is to equip and inspire you and my guidelines are merely suggestions. You do not need to learn them by heart; trust yourself and your ability to give support. Remember that it is your *love* and *presence* that matter the most.

Do not let her pain scare you

Witnessing someone you love and care for in great pain can trigger a lot of emotions. You might get the urge to call in all available midwives and doctors and to inject her with every pain medication possible. You might get stressed, because you do not know what to do or how to help her. It is very important *not* to be afraid of her *pain*. She will need you to be strong and support her more than ever before.

Right there in the eye of the storm, it is crucial that you can take charge for a while and help her to stay on track. You might have to do this even though she says she cannot stand it anymore. It does not necessarily mean that she has given up when she says these things; she might just need to vent her frustration. It sometimes feels good for her to say that she does not want to continue any more, or that she wants pain relief. Very often all that is required is for the people around her to affirm what she is feeling and to guide her to get back on track.

Women in labour sometimes become aggressive, be hard to communicate with, or pull away from your efforts to help her; you need to be there for her regardless of what she says, does or what circumstances arise. Trust your abilities and have faith in your role as a support person. Try not to take what happens personally. Instead, try to see yourself as her most important companion, guide and support.

Step In And Take The Lead

By observing a woman's *body language*, you will clearly see when she has drifted into a negative pattern. If you learn, through the previous chapters, to read the body and its signals during stress and fear, you can then actively interrupt that negative pattern by using the four tools. Be brave and choose to take the lead if you see her getting lost or losing focus. Having the courage to assist someone who is stressed, lost or angry can be a lot harder than you might imagine. You need to be able to express yourself *clearly* and *confidently*; if you don't do it in this way the woman may not follow your guidance.

The guidelines in this part are meant to be a *framework* for you to work with, so that you can make suggestions, whilst at the same time feeling secure and grounded in yourself. You will have the opportunity to gather sentences and techniques that gently direct her back towards trust and confidence, whilst also not disturbing her own techniques. They also give the woman the feeling of being in charge and in control when deciding whether or not she wants the support, or whether she wishes to use the tools. You are never meant to say 'do this' or 'do that'. It is important that you stay sensitive to her needs and that you communicate positively and effectively, physically as well as verbally.

Be brave

It can be difficult to know when, or how to intervene during labour. How firm should you be? What assistance should you offer? How should you act if she cries? What if she resists your help? The labouring woman will need you the most when she feels her power is lacking, her confidence faltering or that she is losing her momentum. This is when you must step in; she needs you to lovingly take over and act as her source of power and faith. She needs to hear: 'You can do this, I am here with you and I will help you get through the next contraction.' To prevent you from standing back when she is struggling, you need to come up with a plan as to how to handle these situations. Agree on how she wants you to guide her, even when she is angry, upset, frustrated, or when she asks for pain relief. When, or if, she reaches a limit and might really need pain medication, you both need to agree on how she can communicate this in a clear way as well.

Encourage and be clear

Pregnant women feel a wide range of emotions leading up to and during childbirth. Fear, anxiety, uncertainty, expectation, anticipation and excitement all flow through her. Decide beforehand how you should react and deal with strong outbursts of emotions. This will make it easier for you to take charge and help her through a particularly difficult phase. The most important thing to remember is to try to highlight the positive. The words 'brave', 'good' or 'fantastic' are effective and encouraging. You might also consider using the word 'dare'. Talk about which words she likes.

> *'I know it feels difficult... but I am here, and I am going to help you. Let's face the next contraction together... here it is... look into my eyes... breathe... now it subsides... let it go... and now rest.'*

> *'You are so relaxed... keep doing what you are doing. Move your body... just like so.'*

> *'You are so brave. Dare to go just a little further, a little further.'*

Humour

Making the woman *laugh* is a great way of helping her. Fear can make her get stuck in negative thoughts and feelings, so laughter can make her look at the situation with a little distance and with a sense of humour. Childbirth is normally full of funny situations and humour is a great tool. You do not have to be a clown, but you can ease an otherwise tense atmosphere by highlighting the funny situations and sounds. Many couples also have a number of familiar in-jokes that can come in handy to lighten a moment. Laughter also boosts oxytocin production, with all its benefits – both for the labouring woman and the support person.

Create a safe environment

The labouring woman needs you as a guide, a coach and a companion. Fear makes her body become tense and hinders the birth process. You need to help her to let go and 'surrender' to her body's process, regardless of whether or not she has any analgesia on board. You also need to create an environment that signals security and safety around her. Your task is to keep an eye on *everything surrounding her* so that she can focus on what is happening *inside* of her. This awareness includes body contact, eye contact, light, sound and everything in your environment, as well as your voice. Do not underestimate the importance of the surrounding and the atmosphere that you create for her.

A doula

If you are the woman's partner, you are of course the *most* important support person and it is great if you feel comfortable being the sole support person. You can also choose to share the task with someone with experience, like a doula or someone else close to you, like a mother or friend.

A doula is a woman with experience of helping labouring women who can give emotional and informational support before, during and immediately after childbirth. The word 'doula' is Greek and means, roughly translated, 'a woman caregiver'. Experienced women have helped other women give birth throughout human history. Since the 1960s births began happening more and more within hospital environments and this has partly led to the important role of the support person for the labouring woman becoming somewhat overlooked.

Having an extra person present does not imply the woman considers her partner to be inept. The doula can never replace the partner, but rather, she represents a calm presence in situations that may be unfamiliar to the partner. Her task is to help create a positive birth experience for the two of you.

Giving birth in the western world is safer today than it has ever been in history, but at the same time, it can also be more stressful and lonelier than ever. The main task of the doula is to protect the birth experience and to guide the labouring woman and her partner by sharing useful tools and techniques for facing the challenges ahead. She supports the birthing woman in whatever decisions she makes and she respects the fact that all women are different and have different needs.

Her task is to remind the partner and nurture the woman through her contractions by using massage, touch and emotional support. As a doula, she does not belong to a specific hospital or team, neither does she have any medical role in the birth process. She is therefore not a substitute for a midwife. She does not usually have a medical degree and her main role consists of emotionally nurturing the labouring woman and her partner throughout the labour, however long it might last. The doula can focus on encouraging and reassuring, without having to worry about anything else. There are many doulas working today, some of them work professionally and others on a voluntary basis.

Practical guidelines for support

8 Principles for support during contractions

1 Lift the hand

To avoid having to guess what the woman wants or if she likes what you are doing, agree in advance *how* you will communicate during the contractions. She needs to feel free, without having to worry about offending or hurting someone's feelings. Simple gestures for 'yes', 'no', and 'stop' are often the most effective. One such gesture might be her raising her hand if something does not feel good.

> *'Lift your hand as soon as it doesn't feel good and I will stop.'*

> *'If you want me to stop, say "Stop." If I talk too much, tell me to be quiet or raise your hand.'*

2 Three contractions

It can be difficult to be brave enough to take over and guide the woman in a different direction if you see that she is struggling. To make this easier, you can ask her to try doing what you suggest for *three contractions*. Remember that the final choice is hers to make; have confidence in yourself and do not take it personally if she does not find your suggestions helpful.

'I will give you a massage. If you find this disturbs you, just lift your hand. Let's try this during three contractions and if it doesn't work, we'll go back to doing it as you were before.'

'I will talk you through the contraction. Lift your hand if you want me to be quiet. Let's try this during three contractions. After that, we can evaluate and see if it made things easier or not.'

❸ From the moment the contraction starts

For you to help a labouring woman, you need to catch her right at the moment she feels the contraction beginning. If you start in the middle of the contraction and she does not have time to follow your instructions, the contraction can easily become too much for her to handle. It is a good idea to use a code word like 'now', or a gesture for when the contraction starts, like raising a hand. That way, you will be right there from the start, guiding her to breathe calmly, getting heavy, using her deep voice and allowing herself to flow with her body.

'Simply say "now" when you feel the contraction coming so that I can help you'

❹ Less is more

We often try to explain ourselves using many words or long sentences. This can disturb the focus of a woman in labour and can also be irritating and confusing. Words are equally as important as touch. They should be clear, simple, few in number and precise. It is also effective to communicate by repeating the *same word* over and over again.

'Remember, heavy... heavy... heavy'.

'Relax your shoulders... relax your jaw... let your body become heavy. Relax your shoulders... relax your jaw... let your body become heavy.'

⑤ Repeat

Get used to sounding like a broken record! Most labouring women need to hear you repeat whatever it is that you are saying an infinite number of times. You might not think she wants to hear 'get heavy' any more after having heard these words for the last three hours. However, if you stop, she might lose her direction and feel discouraged or exasperated. Imagine her stuck in a tornado that she is trying to navigate. The force is enormous and these exact words you repeat can work as her safety harness. Therefore, you should keep talking, maintain your touch and stay close through every contraction.

'Heavy... heavy... heavy. Feel yourself getting heavier... heavy... heavy ... heavy.'

'Lower your shoulders, let them fall, heavy... heavy... heavy... lower your shoulders... heavy, heavy...'

⑥ Do it with her

The woman will not follow your instructions if you simply use just *words* to describe them. She is in the middle of an extremely physical experience, hence she may only be receptive to physical instructions. Therefore, *you* should follow your own instructions. She might not do as you say, but she will *do as you do*. If you want her to use a deep voice, *you* should use a deep voice. If you do this, the woman will have an easier time following your lead automatically, rather than if you simply tell her to 'use a deep voice' without doing it yourself. If you want her to try saying 'yes', *you* should say 'yes', and so on.

> *'You can make as much noise as you like but do it with a deep voice. Do it with me... deep.'*

7 Focus on the moment

Help her remain in the moment, focusing on *one* contraction at a time. Be aware that speaking about *time* has a *negative* effect. Focus on what she has done, and not what she has yet to do.

> *'Let's put this contraction on the pile of all other contractions you have already had.'*

> *'You have made it through all these contractions, and you will never have to do the same ones ever again.'*

8 Quiet time between the contractions.

For a woman to be brave, to go deep into her body and to follow its lead, she will need to have space to focus her attention. You need to whisper and take it slowly in between the contractions so that she can maintain her focus. You could ask, 'Is it okay with you if we talk now? Let us know if we are disturbing you.' A woman's concentration during contractions can be disturbed extremely easily; even the slightest noise or small talk can disrupt her focus. Other women, however, like having chatter in the background. So again, use your communication skills and discern what she wants and what works best for her.

A woman in labour will commonly not be able to talk very much. Nor should she be expected to do so, since she must be able to concentrate and focus completely on the physical work necessary. Therefore, it is important to find other ways to communicate and express yourselves, such as physical closeness, touch, smiles, kisses, cuddles, signs or gestures.

Massage and touch

I was assisting Tina and Joel as a doula. When I arrived, I found Tina all revved up in full motion. She was almost running around in circles and was surprised by the pace and force of the contractions. The fight-or-flight response in her body was obvious; she was constantly moving, her muscles were tense, her gaze kept shifting and her movements were jerky. I approached and softly began to stroke Tina, encouraging her to lean on me, with her head resting on my shoulder. She immediately shifted to a lower gear. We were standing really close to each other, swaying back and forth through a few contractions. The rhythm was slow and soothing and she was resting, letting the contractions come and go. When we had found the rhythm and she was back in tune with her body, her partner Joel took over. They stood close together for a long time. She felt completely safe and present in the moment. The closeness helped her to relax and time passed by more comfortably. After a while she wanted to lie on her side on the bed. Tina was allowing her body to become heavy, being brave, and breathing deeply. Despite this, she found it difficult not to let the tension rise. We started massaging her by stroking our hands from the top of her shoulders, down her back and down to her hips. It relaxed her enough and she managed to rest for a while.

The contractions became more forceful. Tina worked on breathing quietly and feeling heavy. We continued to massage Tina to help her passively follow her body. The midwife arrived and joined us. Joel was right there, close to Tina, massaging and caressing her, encouraging her and showing her that he was right there for her. They stayed in body contact the whole time and the massages kept Tina calm and serene. After a while we could hear that it was time to push and so we helped her kneel on some pillows on the floor. Joel encouraged her, guiding her along, and she managed to follow his prompts and her body's signals. Soon, the head of the baby was visible. Tina was completely relaxed and able to rest in between pushes. Her body had been able to recharge and she had the energy needed to push the baby out. A beautiful girl was born and the mood was calm.

When the birthing woman first encounters pain, her brain reacts by trying to understand and control the sensation. She tries to take charge with her mind and to control the next contraction; how long it will last, the level of pain and how long will the labour go on for? The brain is analysing frantically and a lot of energy is wasted. Since it is impossible to give birth using just your mind and brain, it gets in the way of the body accessing its own natural ability. You can help block this detrimental mental activity by the use of *touch* or *closeness*.

Touch will draw the energy from the brain to the body; the birthing woman will feel heavy and sleepy, she will feel a greater connection to her own body and her mind and thoughts will quieten down. She can slowly relax, forget about time and focus only on the present moment. She cares less about what is happening *outside* of her, instead she is able to serenely settle into her body, fully present. The desire to talk, think and control lose their appeal and she is able to more passively let the wave of the contractions do their work through her body.

This is the reason why massage and touch are such powerful tools for the support person to use in labour. The skin is our biggest sensory organ and *massage* can be a wonderful way of stimulating relaxation, a sense of well-being, strength and inner power. *Touch* releases the hormone *oxytocin*, which has an important role in ensuring the contractions progress the labour, it reduces stress, calms you down and helps desensitise pain during labour. Through massage and touch, the support person can communicate directly with, and influence the actions and responses of, the woman's body in labour.

Oxytocin

Oxytocin is one of the important hormones associated with labour, bonding with the baby and breastfeeding and it is released through touch, warmth, security and calmness. Therefore, it is often called the 'peace and calm' hormone. Oxytocin works against fear and stress and it can help the woman rest and even sleep during the birthing process. It is also a powerful anxiety suppressor. Its most interesting affect however, is that it works beautifully as a pain suppressor as well. The pain gets registered in the brain, however the body's response and reaction to it is turned down.

Gate control theory

Massage works mainly because of the positive effects of oxytocin, however it can also work via the 'gate control theory'. This theory is based on the fact that the sensations from *touch* and *pain* take *different paths* to the brain. If these impulses arrive at the same time, the pain impulses are overridden by the touch impulses by means of a mechanism that gives priority to the touch impulses. The brain perceives a *smaller* number of pain impulses and therefore, the woman experiences *less* pain.

Stay close

Physical contact releases oxytocin, and closeness helps the woman rest during the breaks throughout the childbirth process. Even the short pauses between contractions can be useful if she feels secure and calm; they are great for her to rest or sleep and to gather her strength. The closeness helps her to be brave, not to feel alone and facilitates giving in to the birthing process. It feels good to snuggle up close to someone. It feels safe, and she can relax in a natural and familiar way. Negative emotions are less likely to take over while she can feel someone close by her all the time.

Although the closeness minimises her fight-or-flight responses it does not mean she will automatically feel energised or that she will have enough willpower. It does mean however, that her sense of security is *stronger* than her fear. These feelings may coexist, but the sense of safety she gets from the support person will help her to move forward through the birth journey.

Maintain physical contact with each other throughout the whole labour and birth. This can be an amazing process that will make your bond stronger and your relationship richer and fuller. So, get close to one another! Embrace, hug her and maintain body contact. Show her it is okay to be open and vulnerable. If standing, let her lean as much of her body on you as possible, so that she feels safe and enclosed. Many people also forget that it is okay to kiss during childbirth. Kissing keeps the jaw and mouth relaxed, as well as boosting oxytocin production. Rock and sway during the contractions; this promotes rhythm and relaxation. It is important to sway softly, calmly and slowly. The woman can also sway and rock by herself. I have observed many women while they sway from side to side during contractions, completely present in the moment, massaging their belly with their eyes closed.

The woman can remain close to her support person even if she uses gas and air, an injection of pain relief or an epidural. However, be aware that some women feel uncomfortable and suffocated by closeness. If this is the case, you can still work with verbal support.

Remember to maintain physical contact throughout the *entire* birth process; *do not step back and leave the woman when the staff come in*. Stay close during and between the contractions, especially as their intensity and frequency grows. Hug and hold, and spoon on the bed (even on the birthing bed in the room). Based on the character of your relationship, maintain as much body and skin contact as possible.

Exercise

Snuggle up on the bed or the settee. Cuddle the woman, making sure she is completely wrapped up and relaxed. Try to be as close to each other as possible. Practise having as much of your bodies in contact as possible. Try different positions and see what feels comfortable and good.

Massage techniques during contractions

Basic principles for touch during contractions

Oxytocin is released by a pleasant touch, closeness and comfortable warmth. Therefore, classic massage might not be the most comfortable, as it usually goes deep into the muscle tissue. It is generally better to stroke rhythmically or, squeeze gently. Always massage in a *downward* direction, as this reinforces the direction of the contractions and the downward movement of the baby.

Sometimes the woman does not want to be caressed or touched. My experience, however, is that this has a lot to do with *how* she is touched and *in what way* you have physical contact with her.

Firm Hands with Pressure

Using the tools requires a lot of concentration and the way you touch the labouring woman is important to focus on. A flimsy grip might be perceived as disturbing or annoying. Use confident, firm, steady hands when you touch her. Avoid patting, haphazard or restless movements, nor should you use limp hands. Use pressure.

Maintain a firm pressure or squeeze on different parts of the woman's body through the contraction; this could be on her head, shoulders, arms or legs. Experiment and see what feels good for her and what creates a feeling of security.

The Rhythm of Your Touch
Rhythm is another important aspect of touch. If your touch or your instructions have the wrong rhythm, you might upset and distract, rather than calm and uplift. Let the rhythm be *slow, firm* and *repetitive*.

Flowing Massage
Using the palm of your hand and your fingers straight and *slightly apart*; stroke downwards, from the top of the shoulders to the pelvis, or alternatively from the neck and shoulders down the arms. Use the whole hand, focusing most of the pressure in the fingers. This should be done in one movement and with a firm, steady pressure.

Squeeze Massage
Cup your hand with the *fingers together*, as if compacting a snowball. Squeeze softly and evenly with your hands from the neck, across the shoulders and then down the arms. Then try going from the shoulders down the back, all the way out to the buttocks and thighs. *Squeeze and release, squeeze and release.*

Butterfly Massage
If the pain is strong around the groin and pubic bone, the support person can use a technique called the butterfly massage. This involves a *very light touch*, using the fingertips, like the wings of a

butterfly, to the lower abdomen, back, arms or any other place on the birthing mother's body that feels right for her. The butterfly massage, or 'thousand hand massage' works as a pain inhibitor in accordance with the gate control theory.

The woman can do this herself by standing up and swaying from side to side while tickling her own belly. This is soothing and the tickling will distract from the pain impulses.

Firm Pressure on the Lumbar Region

As labour progresses, the pain will usually move from the lower abdomen to the lower back – the lumbar region. Light touch and massage work very well on the lower abdomen, however the back needs more force, so use more pressure when massaging this area. For some women, the pain of the contractions can be felt primarily in the back from the beginning of labour.

The best technique is to use is small, *circular* massage, using quite a bit of force, at the base of the spine, just above the buttocks. Use the lower part of the palm of your hand or the fingertips of your four closed fingers (i.e. not using the thumb). This massage helps to block the pain signals.

Brief overview

BREATHING

What is important is breathing *softly* and *quietly* throughout the entire contraction, one contraction at a time.

Role of the Support Person:

The breathing should be soft, slow and quiet
The instruction 'quietly' will help you to continuously guide the woman towards the most effective breathing. As soon as you can *hear* her breath, you step in and encourage her to go *softer* and *quieter*.

> *'Breathe in soooftly, quietly … slooowly breathe out … Breathe in soooftly, quietly … slooowly, quietly breathe out.'*

If she struggles with the *slow* breathing, guide her towards a faster rhythm, but keep it *quiet*. Try and ensure that the breathing is *quiet* and *soft*, since it often remains audible despite the instruction. You might think to yourself, 'Well, it is almost soundless, and she seems to be doing okay.' However, try to encourage her to breathe *without* sound during at least *three contractions* to see the difference. It is worth it, I promise!

Establish how you will communicate together

This is so that you will know immediately each contraction begins and will be able to help her from the beginning. She may raise her hand or say 'now' as soon as she feels the first sign of a new contraction.

'Say "now" or raise your hand as soon as you feel the contraction so that I can help you.'

Finish the contraction with a sigh

Encourage her to finish every contraction by taking a deep breath in, followed by a big sigh as she breathes out. This will release any tension that has built up during the contraction.

'The contraction is over. Fill your lungs with air and let's exhale with a soft and lovely sigh together [sigh with her].'
'Sigh the air out and let any tension melt away.'

Remember the strength of repetition

This involves repeating the same simple but powerful words, reminding her of the quiet breathing, and as each contraction wears off, you remind her of the sigh, and so on. During each contraction you keep repeating your instructions calmly and deeply over and over again.

🔩 RELAXATION

When the birthing woman feels the contraction come, she needs to let go of her whole body; face, jaw, shoulders, bottom and thighs. Explore and try different positions, such as standing, lying down on the right or left side, or walking. Imagining the body sinking into water can be a powerful visual aid.

Role of the Support Person;

Encouraging 'heavy', soft, relaxed muscles
As the contraction starts, you should help the woman to become 'heavy' in her body. She should be like a rag doll, letting go of all tension.

> *'The contraction is coming. Be still and lean on me. Let go and let everything sink down.'*

Help the woman to let go and become heavy in her *jaw, shoulders, bottom* and *thighs*. Use simple words while guiding her. You might find the word 'heavy' or 'down' useful. Direct her with a calm, deep voice.

> *'Relax your jaw... release your shoulders... heavy bottom and legs... relax your jaw... release your shoulders... heavy bottom and legs...'*

Repeat this over and over again. Try to see *where* she holds tension and bring her attention to these areas. Stroke her jaw, shoulders and brow if you see any tension there. Do this repeatedly. If you see a frown on her forehead, lovingly and gently sweep your thumb or fingertips across this area, while repeating…

'Relax your forehead… smooth face… heavy…'

The 'simplicity principle'
Establish the 'simplicity principle' by choosing to repeat phrases or words over and over again, using a calm, deep voice.

'Relax your jaw, let go of your shoulders, feel your weight, heavy, heavy, heavy.'

👄 THE VOICE

There are benefits from the woman using a *deep* voice that resonates from the lower abdomen. The sound should be smooth and audible throughout the entire exhalation. In the pushing stage of labour, it can be a good idea to close the mouth and let the sound resonate within. Do not be afraid or embarrassed of making sounds!

Role of the Support Person:

Help the woman find her deep, low-pitched voice
Making an 'aaaahhhh' or 'mmmmm' sound with slightly open or closed lips can help at the end of the first stage when the contractions become more intense.

In the second stage of labour, gently closing the mouth and making an 'mmmmmmmm' sound will engage the muscles she needs to push. It is helpful to show the way with your own voice to demonstrate how the tone should be slow and deep.

'Make as much noise as you want, as long as you use a deeeeep voice. Lower and deeper. Let the voice go all the way down to your belly. Deeep... deeep... deep.'

Words for the pushing stage

When she is in the pushing phase, you can help her feel heavy and sink towards her heels if she is kneeling or on all fours, or alternatively towards the floor or down into the bed. Repeat the word 'down'. 'Brave' and 'dare' are also words that work wonderfully well when it comes to encouraging her to do just that – to dare to try different things and to be brave.

'Dare to sink towards your heels. Only think about the word down... down... down... down... you are so brave...'

She will 'mirror' what you do

She will find it much easier and more effective to copy, or 'mirror', what you do, rather than to do as you say. So, she will tend to copy your breathing pattern for example, and if you use a deep, low voice she is likely to try doing the same.

THE MIND

If you feel that negative energy or thoughts are starting to take over, there is power in starting to say 'yes'. It needs to be said slowly, repeatedly, using a calm, deep voice.

The Role of the Support Person:

Dealing with negative emotions

If the negative emotions gets too strong, or if she starts saying 'no', you can help her by saying 'yes' in your own calm, deep voice. Applying humour at this point is also a good idea. This could be a common thread through the entire birth process; use your sense of humour and fun to make her laugh, smile and relax.

> 'Dare to say 'yes' instead of 'no'. During the next three contractions try saying 'yes'... you do not have to continue if it doesn't feel right. Yeeeeesss... follow along... yeeeess... yeeess...'

The power of three contractions

Suggest she tries any change or something new for *three contractions*. More than this can feel overwhelming, but trying something over three contractions is manageable and often opens up new ways of coping with the contractions.

Use of touch and massage as a birth partner
You can use touch and massage in order to reinforce the tools and to reduce stress and anxiety. Remember that massage and touch help block some of the pain signals that go to the brain, hence lessening the sensations of pain. It also helps the woman to relax, softens the muscles and leads to a more positive experience of labour and birth.

Techniques

Massage or stroke by starting at the shoulders and slowly and firmly bringing your hands down along her back, on either side of her spine, to the top of the buttocks, and continue down the sides of the upper thighs if you wish. Alternatively, start at the back of the neck and go across the shoulders and down the arms. You might also want to include foot massage in your repertoire, since this is highly effective.

1. Stay close and use a firm, still hand with pressure.

2. Keep your hands stretched open, with fingers slightly apart. Massage slowly and firmly, applying most pressure with your fingers. Make it one long, calm and sweeping movement.

3. Cup your hands slightly, with your fingers together. Massage by squeezing one part of her body after another, moving your hands one inch at a time. Start by massaging the neck, then move across the shoulders and down her arms.

4. In case you do not like any of these techniques – create your own way of massaging. Whichever technique you find useful, remember that the movement should be from the top and going *downwards*, whether it be her arms, back or thighs.

5. Observe where the woman is holding tension – the forehead, jaw, shoulders, hands? Then massage or stroke those areas.

6. Remember to speak with a soft, deep voice and remind her to breathe softly and quietly.

'Let your shoulders drop, relax your entire back. [massage gently]'

Butterfly massage

If the woman's lower abdomen and top of her legs are aching, you can massage this area using a light touch, like a butterfly. Use the fingertips from just above the pubic bone, above the pubic hair and along the fold where the abdomen joins the inner, upper thighs.

You can also do this across the whole belly with sweeping motions. Ask her what feels best.

Firm pressure to the lumbar region

When the pain gets strong in the woman's back, you can massage her sacrum; this is the bony area you can feel in the lower back, just above the buttocks. You can use varied pressure, although women often like a very firm, circular motion and pressure. See what works best.

At the same time as you apply pressure to her lower back, remind her to breathe through her whole body, to become 'heavy' and to relax her shoulders and jaw.

In some cases, the woman is sensitive towards pressure and finds it uncomfortable. If this is the case, you can use the softer techniques instead.

Key Points for the Woman in Labour

Does all of this feel a bit complicated? Please do not worry. At the end of the day, all you have to remember when each contraction starts is;

1. Breathe *quietly* to the rhythm of your choice when the contraction comes. As it subsides, exhale with one or two soft and audible *sighs*.

2. During the contraction, relax your *face, jaw, shoulders* and *buttocks,* while letting your body sink heavily towards the floor.

3. As the birth process gets towards the pushing phase, you can greet the contractions with a deep voice and the feeling of being 'heavy'.

4. If you feel that negative thoughts are beginning to take over and you have a hard time carrying on, use the word 'yes'. Repeat the word softly, calmly and with a deep voice throughout the contraction.

5. If you wish, your support person can give you a massage with a *slow, firm, rhythmical* touch and with a *downward* movement, which will give you a sense of security and closeness.

To download the summary sheet and to access our in depth training together with your suport person visit

www.birthbyheart.com

Conclusion

I have now shown you how fear can be the biggest obstacle you have to face in labour, but also how by using simple tools, you can dare to face this fear and transform your birth experience. I have shown you that you have an inner power, and how specific tools will help your body unlock the systems you already possess to help you give birth.

But all this will not lead to the perfect birth, because the perfect birth does not really exist! Childbirth is a process where every step is important and where every emotion is true. Just like life itself, the process can be an emotional rollercoaster ride; you will have faith, you will lose faith, and then you will regain faith again. Ideals and perfection do not belong in the birthing room. Preconceived ideas about having the perfect, natural birth, or alternatively having a highly medicated birth without a trace of pain, can both have a negative effect on you. Such preconceptions are equally restrictive and limiting, since they are not based on humility and respect for the process and the person you are.

Childbirth encompasses your whole being; your worst, as well as your best, self. Giving birth to a baby carries with it an opportunity to conquer obstacles within, such as low self-esteem, lack of trust in your body's abilities, or a hidden lack of trust in yourself. This involves facing up to your deepest fears and all your doubts. If you understand how childbirth harbours your whole being and everything you carry with you, you have the opportunity to face up to these things and heal them. Every step is yours to take, and every step is important. You decide what is best for you, depending on how you feel at the time. There is no right or wrong way of doing things or giving birth; the focus should be on trusting that you can *grow* from the experience, and that you can birth your baby.

Many women believe that they will emerge with a mainly positive experience of pain because they have prepared themselves before giving birth. This can leave them feeling disappointed if they have a hard time during labour, or struggle to cope with the pain they experience. They struggle to find the meaning in what they are doing; they can feel the experience is empty and futile. I had that same feeling during my first labour, until I got the support that enabled me to move through the course of events, and ultimately to access my body's abilities. I was not able to fully comprehend and make sense of what had happened until after the birth. Then, I was able to learn and grow from the experience. Therefore, as an important part of mental preparation, it is vital to keep in mind how the reward for what you are doing might not come right away, as you are doing it, but instead can come later.

Childbirth can be divided into two parts. The first part is when you enter the birth and, through hard work, grant the body access to itself. Here, you do not know why you do what you do; you simply do it. It is like running a marathon or climbing a mountain, where you move forward one breath at a time, inch by inch, along with your partner or support person. As you choose to take the next step, you focus on carrying on, without resisting what your body is trying to do and for which it is designed.

It is not until you have reached the other side of the mountain, or the finishing line, that you will be able to make sense of your struggles and challenges. This second part of childbirth is when you will reap the benefits; your innermost boundaries have been stretched and your horizon has forever widened. After you have given birth, in whatever way it may have occurred, your consciousness will start to understand, interpret and make sense of what happened. For many women, this leads to higher self-esteem, a better capacity to embrace life and a new way of appreciating their own bodies.

The most important thing to keep with you is something a woman once said to me; 'Childbirth is but a whisper of all the challenges you will face afterwards. When you begin nurturing a growing, developing child and all the wonderful trials and blessings that brings… that is when it truly begins!'

Good luck!
With Love! Susanna Heli

Thank you

There are so many women and men who have guided me to the place where I am today, and especially the women whose births I have had the honour of witnessing. They taught me all I know, and they showed me when I did something right and when I did something wrong. For this, I am deeply grateful.

A midwife who has been of great importance in helping me find my inner powers is *Cayenne Ekjordh*. You led me towards my inner voice and wisdom. Your immense intuition and ability to know what I, and other birthing women, need to be able to channel in order to have an empowering experience, has inspired me greatly. I am eternally grateful! You also taught me the invaluable 'diving technique', upon which I have based many of my tools.

I also want to thank midwife *Gudrun Abascal* for her exceptional support during my years as an assisting nurse, when I explored and experimented at BB-Stockholm, a maternity ward in Sweden. Your unyielding belief in putting the woman first and letting everyone around her protect her in different ways has helped me to develop.

Thank you, *Mariano Amarilla*, for all your help in structuring and developing this book. Without you, nobody would have understood anything I was trying to say. Your competence is endless! Even though I did not always jump for joy when you pulled parts of what I had written to pieces, I will always be infinitely thankful. You are just as much a part of the creation of this book as I am.

Thank you to *Liisa Svensson,* who has helped me with the book and my ability to grow both as a doula and as a human being. The unique linguistic talents of *Viktoria Wallin*, *Hilda Lundgren* and *Eugénia Hildestrand* have helped me express myself better, using my own words. You showed me where I needed to expand and elaborate. You have inspired, elevated and broadened my language. My sister, *Heidi Karikumpu*, and *Fatima Durrani*, represented the link between myself and my readers. Your courage in asking me what I wanted to say, or letting me know when you did not understand, helped me to not 'muddle things' nor use unintelligible words. In a clear and uncomplicated way, you helped me keep track of, and keep hold of, the common thread.

Thank you, *Christina Lundberg*, *Iréne Setterqvist* and *Sofia Jansson* who, through their extensive experience and wisdom, continues to develop the method continually alongside me. I also want to send out a big 'thank you' to all the people who are part of the 'Birth Without Fear method'; thank you to all instructors and co-workers. An extra thank you to Emilie Wicks and Alison Sethna for helping me with the English edition and putting your love into the words and content. Thank you also to *Kerstin Uvnäs Moberg*, whose influence in the creation and development of the method cannot be understated. I am so fortunate to be able to call you my friend and to learn from your deep wisdom.

Many thanks to all the women and couples who have read the book – this venture would not be possible without you.

Last, but not least, many thanks to all the *midwives* and maternity *nurses* who have shown me invaluable techniques to use during labour. I have had so much fun sharing the births with you. I want to also specifically thank the staff at BB-Stockholm.

Forever grateful!
Susanna Heli

References

The Birth Without Fear method
www.birthbyheart.com

- Abascal, G. Att föda (2004). Albert Bonniers Förlag.
- Alehagen, S. Fear, Pain and Stress Hormones During Labor (2002). Magisteruppsats i Linköping, University Medical Dissertations No. 730, PMID 16295513.
- Antonovsky, A. Hälsans mysterium (1991). Natur och Kultur, Sweden.
- Balaskas, J. New Active Birth: A Concise Guide to Natural Childbirth (1991). Thorsons.
- Brudal, L. Födandets psykologi (1985). Natur och Kultur.
- England, P. & Horowits, R. Birthing From Within (1998). Partera Press.
- Gaskin, I.M. Ina May's Guide To Childbirth (2003). Bantam Dell.
- Dick-Read, G. Childbirth Without Fear (2012). Pinter & Martin.
- Gronlien Zetterqvist, K. Att vara kroppssubjekt: Ett fenomenologiskt bidrag till feministisk teori och religionsfilosofi (2002). Studia Philosophiae Religionis 23.
- Heiberg-Endresen, E. & Björnstad, N. Fødende krefter (1992). J.W. Cappelens Förlag.

- Kitzinger, S. The New Pregnancy & Childbirth (2008). Dorling Kindersley.
- Klaus, M.H., Kennell, J.H. & Klaus, P.H. Mothering the Mother (1996). Addison-Wesley.
- Kåver, A. Att leva ett liv, inte vinna ett krig (2007). Natur och Kultur.
- Lerner, M. Psykosomatik, kroppens och själens dialog (1999). Natur och CB_4.9.12_final.indd 188 13/09/2012 15:59 Kultur.
- Lundberg, U. & Wentz, G. Stressad hjärna, stressad kropp: Om sambandet mellan psykisk stress och kroppslig ohälsa (2005). Wahlström & Widstrand.
- Lännergren, J. m.fl. Fysiologi (1998). Studentlitteratur.
- Nisell, R. & Lundberg, T. Smärta och inflammation: Fysiologi och terapi vid smärttillstånd i rörelseorganen (1999). Studentlitteratur.
- O'Driscoll, K. & Meagher D. Active Management of Labor (1993). Mosby.
- Simkin, P. The Birth Partner (1989). The Harvard Common Press.
- Sjögren, B. Förlossningsrädsla (1998). Studentlitteratur.
- Uvnäs Moberg, K. The Oxytocin Factor (2011). Pinter & Martin.
- Waldenström, U. Föda barn: Från naturligt till högteknologiskt (2007). Karolinska Institutet University Press.
- Währborg, P. Stress och den nya ohälsan (2003). Natur och Kultur. articles

- Alehagen, S., Wijma, B. & Wijma, K. Fear of childbirth before, during and after childbirth. Acta Obstet Gynecol Scand, 2006;85:56–62.
- Alehagen, S. & Wijma, K. & Wijma, B. Fear during labor. Acta Obstet Gynecol Scand, 2001;80:315–320.
- Alehagen, S. m.fl. Fear, pain and stress hormones during childbirth. J Psychosom Obstet Gynaecol, 2005;26:3:153–165.
- Areskog, B., Uddenberg, N. & Kjessler, B. Fear of childbirth in late pregnancy. Gynecol Obstet Invest, 1981;12:262–266.
- Dahlberg, K. Kroppen – vår tillgång till världen. Nord Fysio, 1997;1:29–33.
- Eysenck, M.W. Anxiety, the cognitive perspective. Essays in Cognitive Psychology, 1992:35–50.
- Green, J.M., Coupland, V.A. & Kitzinger, J.V. Expectations, experiences, and psychological outcomes of childbirth: a prospective study of 825 women. Birth, 1990;17:15–24. CB_4.9.12_final.indd 189 13/09/2012 15:59
- Green, J.M. Expectations and experiences of pain in labor: findings from a large prospective study. Birth, 1993;20:65–72.
- Hedlund, L. & Gard, G. Tillit till den egna kroppen. Nord Fysio, 2000;4:67–74.
- Henry, J.P. Biological basis of the stress response. Integr Physiol Behav Sci, 1992;1:66–83.

- Hodnet, E.D. m.fl. Continuous support for women during childbirth Cochrane Database of Systematic Reviews, 2007:3, Art. No. CDOO3766.DOI: 10.1002/14651858. CDOO3766.pub2.
- Hodnet, E.D. m.fl. Continuous support for women during childbirth Cochrane Database of Systematic Rewiews, 2007:3, Art. No. CDOO3766 DOI: 10.1002/14651858. CDOO3766.pub2.
- Kennedy, H.P. m.fl. The landscape of caring for women: A narrative study of midwifery practice. Journal of Midwifery and Women's Health, 2004 Jan–Feb;49(1):14–23, PMID 14710136.
- Lagercrantz, H. & Slotkin, T.A. The 'stress' of being born. Scientific American, 1985;12:100–110.
- Lederman, R.P. m.fl. Anxiety and epinephrine in multiparous women in labor. Relationship to duration of labor and fetal heart rate pattern. J Psychosom Obstet Gynaecol, 1985;153:870–877.
- Lovallo, W.R. & Thomas, T.L. Stress hormones in psychophysiological research: Emotional behavioral, and cognitive implications. Handbook of Psychophysiology, Cambridge University Press, 1989:12–33.
- Lowe, N.K. Explaining the pain of active labor: the importance of maternal confidence. Res Nurs Health, 1989;12:237–245.
- McCrea, B.H. & Wright, M.E. & Myrphy-Black, T. Differences in midwifes' approach to pain relief in labor. Midwifery, 1998;14:174–180.

- Melender, H.L. Experiences of fears associated with pregnancy and childbirth: a study of 329 pregnant women. Birth, 2002;29(2):101–111.
- Melzack, R. m.fl. Labor is still painful after prepared childbirth training. Can Med Ass J 1981;25:357–363. CB_4.9.12_final.indd 190 13/09/2012 15:59
- Molin, C. & Nilsson, C.G. Stress – reaktioner och beteende Tandläkartidningen, 1997;89:7.
- Saisto, T. & Halmesmäki, E. Fear of childbirth: a neglected dilemma. Acta Obstet Gynecol Scand, 2003;82:201–208.
- Saisto, T. m.fl. Reduced pain tolerance during and after pregnancy in women suffering from fear of labor. Pain 93, 2001:123–127.
- Simkin, P. Stress, pain and catecholamines in labor: Part 1. A review. Birth, 1986;13:227–233.
- Sjögren, B. Fear of childbirth and psychosomatic support. Acta Obstet Gynecol Scand, 1998;77:819–25.
- Slade, P. Expectations, experiences and satisfaction with labour. Br J Clin psychol. 1993;32:469-83.
- Szeverenyi, P. m.fl. Contents of childbirth-related fear among couples wishing the partner's presence at delivery. J Psychosom Obstet Gynaecol, 1998;19:38–43.
- Thomassen, P. m.fl. Doula – ett nytt begrepp inom förlossnings vården Läkartidningen 2003;51-52:4268–4271.
- Thorstensson, S. & Nissen, E. & Ekstrom, A. An exploration and descriptio of student midwives' experiences in offering continuous labour support to women/couples. Midwifery, 2007 Sep17, PMID 17881100.

- Waldenström, U. & Berman, V. & Vasell, G. The complexity of labor pain: experiences of 278 women. J Psychosom Obstet Gynaecol, 1996b;17:215–228.
- Waldenström, U. Experience of labor and birth in 1111 women. J Psychosom Res, 1999;47:471–82.
- Waldenström, U. m.fl. The childbirth experience, Birth, 1996;23:144–153.
- Zhang, J. m.fl. Continous labor support from labor attendant for primiparous women: A meta-analysis. Obstet Gynaecol, 1996;88:739–744.

Made in the USA
Monee, IL
29 July 2022

.10524389R10122